Secrets of Success:
Getting into Foundation Training

Secrets of Success: Getting into Foundation Training

Edited by

Marc A Gladman PhD, MRCOG, MRCS(Eng), FRCS(Gen Surg)

UKCRC Clinical Lecturer in Surgery, Centre for Academic Surgery, Institute of Cell and Molecular Science, Barts and The London School of Medicine and Dentistry, London, UK

Manoj Ramachandran BSc(Hons), MBBS(Hons), MRCS(Eng), FRCS(Tr&Orth)

Consultant Trauma and Orthopaedic Surgeon, Barts and The London NHS Trust, London, and Honorary Senior Lecturer, William Harvey Research Institute, Barts and The London School of Medicine and Dentistry, London, UK

Mark J Portou MBChB(Hons)

ST2 in Surgery-in-General, London Deanery, London, UK

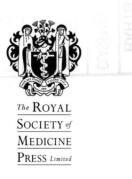

The ROYAL
SOCIETY *of*
MEDICINE
PRESS *Limited*

Published by the Royal Society of Medicine Press Ltd
1 Wimpole Street, London W1G 0AE, UK
Tel: +44 (0)20 7290 2921
Fax: +44 (0)20 7290 2929
Email: publishing@rsm.ac.uk
Website: www.rsmpress.co.uk

British Library Cataloguing in Publication Data
A catalogue record for this book is available from the British Library

ISBN 978-1-85315-886-5

Distribution in Europe and Rest of World:
Marston Book Services Ltd
PO Box 269, Abingdon
Oxon OX14 4YN, UK
Tel: +44 (0)1235 465500
Fax: +44 (0)1235 465555
Email: direct.order@marston.co.uk

Distribution in the USA and Canada:
Royal Society of Medicine Press Ltd
c/o BookMasters Inc
30 Amberwood Parkway
Ashland, OH 44805, USA
Tel: +1 800 247 6553/+1 800 266 5564
Fax: +1 419 281 6883
Email: order@bookmasters.com

Distribution in Australia and New Zealand:
Elsevier Australia
30–52 Smidmore Street
Marrickville NSW 2204, Australia
Tel: +61 2 9517 8999
Fax: +61 2 9517 2249
Email: service@elsevier.com.au

Typeset by Phoenix Photosetting, Chatham, Kent
Printed in the UK by Bell & Bain Ltd, Glasgow

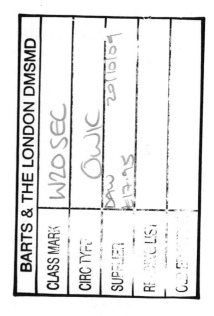

Contents

Contributors

Marc A Gladman PhD, MRCOG, MRCS(Eng), FRCS(Gen Surg)
UKCRC Clinical Lecturer in Surgery, Centre for Academic Surgery,
Institute of Cell & Molecular Science, Barts and The London School
of Medicine & Dentistry, London

Manoj Ramachandran BSc(Hons), MBBS(Hons), MRCS(Eng),
FRCS(Tr&Orth)
Consultant Trauma and Orthopaedic Surgeon, Barts and The London
NHS Trust, London, and Honorary Senior Lecturer, William Harvey
Research Institute, Barts and The London School of Medicine &
Dentistry, London

Mark J Portou MBChB(Hons)
ST2 in Surgery-in-General, London Deanery

Jasdeep K Gill MBChB(Hons)
Academic Foundation Doctor, Hammersmith Hospital, London

Shalini Kawar MBBS, BSc, DRCOG
Specialty Trainee in General Practice, Whipps Cross University
Hospital, Leytonstone, London

Sukhjinder S Nijjer MBChB(Hons), BSc, MRCP
Specialist Registrar in Cardiology, The Royal Brompton Hospital,
London

Elena Nikiphorou MBBS, BSc, MRCP
ST3 in Rheumatology, Eastern Deanery

Philip J Smith BMedSci(Hons), MBBS, MRCP(London)
Academic Clinical Fellow/ST3 in Gastroenterology, University College
London and London Deanery

Shondipon Laha BM, BCh, MA, FRCA
Consultant in Anaesthesia and Critical Care Medicine, Lancashire
Teaching Hospitals NHS Foundation Trust

The philosophy of 'Maximize *Your* Medical Career'

It is now over 15 years since we first met at medical school, united by a passion for education and a desire to excel in our medical careers. During this time we have been working together and have actively designed and delivered numerous products to facilitate the development of medical students and junior doctors. To this day, we are surprised by the lack of formal career guidance and development available to doctors. Professional development for doctors is complex, involving the acquisition of numerous clinical and non-clinical skills. Some individuals are fortunate enough to encounter altruistic peers or senior colleagues who act as mentors; providing informal instruction based on their own experiences. Frequently, however, it is a process of chance or self-tuition for the majority of doctors, some of whom never acquire the necessary skills, particularly non-clinical ones (e.g. succeeding in job applications, leadership, motivation, team working).

The concept of 'Maximize *Your* Medical Career' has been developed by us specifically to address the void in the development of medical students and junior doctors. Our aim is to provide mentorship, comprehensive guidance, and professional development for individual doctors, to facilitate career progression through a portfolio of innovative products that reflect our enthusiasm, energy, and unique style. We hope that you and your future careers can benefit from the knowledge of our own experiences. All too often, we are told to aim to achieve 'competence' in medicine. Our philosophy is never to be satisfied with settling for this, but instead we urge you to strive for 'excellence' and being the best that you can possibly be!

The 'Secrets of Success' series of books embodies this philosophy. The first instalment is aimed at helping you secure your first medical job, which we hope will be the first of many in your future career in medicine.

Marc A Gladman and Manoj Ramachandran
Series Editors

Preface

This book is intended for use by all those applying to the UK Foundation Programme. Medical school should prepare you for life as a junior doctor, but surprisingly little focus is placed on that crucial final hurdle of getting a job. The aim of this text is to address this obvious omission from the undergraduate curriculum. The book is written specifically to guide you through all stages of the online application process. Contained within are both general strategies in relation to the application form and specific guidance covering all the questions on recent application forms. It must be stressed that the aim of this book is not to provide a set of 'perfect' responses to every possible question that may be encountered on application forms for the Foundation Programme. Rather, it aims to teach you certain skills – the tools that you will require to complete your own application successfully, when the time comes. Allied to this point, *we urge you not to be tempted to copy or modify any of the examples included in this book when completing your own application.* Not only is plagiarism a serious offence, but you will have completely missed the point of this book if you intend to use it for that purpose. Further, you will face serious consequences if caught – *you have been warned!*

We have opted for a workbook style for this text, to encourage you to build an individualized collection of examples and experiences that you can draw upon when constructing your own answers for the application form. In addition, the text will teach you to plan and think about your answers, using a logical and systematic approach. Throughout the book, we have used icons to indicate 'Top Tips', 'Danger' areas, 'Ask the Expert', and so on. Look out for these to help you successfully complete your form.

Never before has the postgraduate medical job market been so competitive. Getting an early advantage is therefore essential. This book contains everything that a conscientious applicant will need to succeed.

Good luck!

MAG, MR, MJP

Acknowledgements

We should like to offer our most sincere thanks to everyone at RSM Press Ltd who has supported this project, particularly Sarah Burrows, Sarah Vasey, and Peter Richardson. We also are most grateful to Dr Elizabeth Owen, Specialty Trainee in Paediatrics, for her help proofreading the manuscript. Most importantly, we are grateful to the many medical students and junior doctors whom we have taught over the years for providing feedback that has enabled us to constantly refine and improve our products.

Key for icons

 Top Tip

 Question

 Homework

 Facts and Figures

 Danger

Ask the Expert

1 The Foundation Programme

Mark J Portou

Modernizing Medical Careers: conception of the Foundation Programme

Modernizing Medical Careers (MMC), introduced from 2005 onwards, represented the biggest change in the UK medical postgraduate career and training structure since 1995 and was perhaps the most radical change ever imposed on medical training. Before MMC, training in the UK was based around an 'apprenticeship model'. In this model, a newly qualified doctor would commence work as a pre-registration house officer (PRHO) for 1 year. This year consisted of two 6-month posts (one medical and one surgical), often completed in different hospitals. Appointment to such posts was usually performed by individual medical schools, using 'matching programmes' or occasionally a more formal application process. Satisfactory completion of both posts led to full registration with the General Medical Council (GMC). This process involved no formal assessment of progress; it was often simply a case of keeping the consultant happy so that he or she would sign off the junior doctor at the end of the job!

MMC was devised to address the problems encountered by senior house officers, which were highlighted in the 2002 report by the Chief Medical Officer for England, *Unfinished Business: Proposals for Reform of the Senior House Offer Grade*. A complete change to the structure of postgraduate medical education was recommended, to ensure smooth and integrated progression through the training grades. For the first time, the use of a standardized curriculum was suggested. Robust and consistent tools would be used to assess progress. Further, the selection process was to be overhauled, by creating a national, centralized application procedure.

The Foundation Programme was established as part of this major reform of postgraduate medical education and training. Reform was driven by the need for care to be based on more effective teamwork, a multidisciplinary approach and more flexible training pathways, tailored to meet service and personal development needs. It also reflected the contemporary philosophy that, in the future, patient care would be provided by trained doctors and recognized that existing training systems fell short of this purpose. Training in the UK also needed to be brought more in line with best practice in other countries. Above all, the driver for change was the need for better care systems for patients. Modern training was to be set within effectively managed, quality-assured training programmes compatible with the European Working Time Directive.

The Foundation Programme

The UK Foundation Programme is a 2-year generic training programme designed to bridge the gap between undergraduate and specialist medical training. It builds on undergraduate training to allow Foundation doctors to demonstrate performance in the workplace rather than competence in isolated test situations. Foundation doctors are encouraged to develop clinical thinking and professional judgement, especially where there is clinical uncertainty. Foundation year 1 (F1) expands upon the knowledge, skills and competences learnt at medical school. The curriculum for this year is set by the GMC, and F1 doctors are required to achieve specific competences by the end of this year in order to obtain full registration, which is available to them on completion of F1.

Foundation year 2 (F2) aims to continue this generic experience/ education, building on the skills and competences learnt in F1. The educational focus of F2 is more in the assessment and management of the acutely ill patient, and generic professional skills (teamwork and leadership; time management; communication skills). F2 also provides trainees with the opportunity to experience specialties not previously available to junior grades, such as microbiology, biochemistry, histopathology, public health, and psychiatry. At the end of F2, doctors should be ready to enter a specialty training programme.

Since 2005, all UK medical school graduates have entered the 2-year Foundation Programme, and have participated in its revolutionary ideals of competency-based training, against a standardized national curriculum.

The Tooke inquiry

Following the highly publicized failure of the Medical Training Application Service (MTAS), the online system introduced under MMC in 2007, the Health Secretary in April that year set up an independent inquiry under the chairmanship of Sir John Tooke. An interim report was published in October 2007 and the final report was published in January 2008. The inquiry made 47 recommendations, which, if adopted, will once again have dramatic consequences for the structure of postgraduate medical education. One of these recommendations in particular may affect the Foundation Programme. In his report, Sir John Tooke recommends that the Foundation years should be 'uncoupled'. If accepted, this will mean that F1 will essentially continue unchanged but that F2 will be incorporated into 'Core Training Programmes'. This measure would satisfy UK employment laws while allowing universities to guarantee UK medical graduates a job directly from medical school.

To allay fears regarding the level of experience of newly registered doctors, in comparison with their PRHO counterparts of old, it is recommended that closer integration between the final year of medical school and F1 occurs.

At the time of writing, the Department of Health has accepted some of the Tooke report proposals and delayed making decisions on others, including reform to the Foundation Programme, until after 2010. The Foundation Programme will, therefore, essentially continue in its current form for some years to come.

Registration with the General Medical Council

The F1 year, as previously mentioned, precedes full registration with the GMC. GMC registration is a legal requirement for all medical practitioners in the UK. It confers on the practitioner a licence to prescribe prescription-only medicines, the ability to sign statutory documents such as death certificates, and many responsibilities enshrined in various different acts of UK legislation. The F1 doctor is required to satisfy certain standards set by the GMC in order to achieve full registration, and thus the ability to practise, including being able to prescribe unsupervised.

Provisional registration is obtained in several ways. Graduates from a UK medical school recognized under the Medical Act 1983 are given provisional registration. Doctors qualifying from countries outside the European Union and who have passed the examination of the Professional and Linguistic Assessment Board (PLAB), but who have not completed an internship, are able to apply for provisional registration. Doctors qualifying from countries in the European Union, regardless of where their primary medical qualification was achieved, are also entitled to provisional registration. Provisional registration limits the doctor to F1 posts, and thus full registration is essential for career progression.

The curriculum of the Foundation Programme

Competence-based training is one of the innovations of the Foundation Programme. Previously, postgraduate medical training was delivered on a time-based model. Doctors in training had no defined educational (or career) pathway, no formalized educational goals, and no objective end-point to their training. Further, no formal career support or appraisal system existed. In 2004, an independent body, the Postgraduate Medical Education and Training Board (PMETB), was established to set and oversee the implementation of standards for postgraduate medical education. The PMETB is due to merge with the GMC following the recommendations of the Tooke report.

Foundation Programme doctors now work within approved and scrutinized posts. For the first time, a nationally implemented curriculum exists, which all trainees are expected to follow. With the development of explicit standards against which trainees are measured, more objective and robust assessment tools have emerged with which to evaluate their competence.

Assessment tools of the Foundation Programme

All doctors in training have to show that they have achieved the required level of competence to progress to the next level of training. You have to continuously collect evidence of your progress, keep a portfolio of your achievements, and undergo regular appraisal with an educational supervisor. Sufficient evidence of acquisition of F1 competences is required for you to obtain full GMC registration, and evidence of your attainment of both F1 and 2 competences is required to complete Foundation Programme training.

The assessment tools that you encounter in the Foundation Programme are designed to measure your competence in all aspects of the curriculum, such as specific clinical skills, history taking and examination, communication skills, use and interpretation of investigations, and patient management. The assessments compare your performance against the standard expected of a doctor at the end of your particular year of training. Accordingly, there should be a progression as more experience is gained throughout the year. These assessment tools are intended to be used in the day to day practice of Foundation doctors, and are known collectively as workplace-based assessments.

Workplace-based assessments

The workplace-based assessments form the basis for demonstrating competence. The associated paperwork will be contained in your portfolio, which will be reviewed by your educational supervisor in regular appraisal meetings. These meetings will need to be arranged at the beginning, middle and end of every placement, so that your progression can be monitored.

Three types of assessment are commonly used.

1. Direct observation of doctor–patient interactions

Two forms of direct observation tools are in use:

- Mini-Clinical Evaluation Exercise (Mini-CEX)
- Direct Observation of Procedural Skills (DOPS).

Your performance in a particular situation, for example using a procedural skill (DOPS) or a clinical encounter (Mini-CEX), is observed by a more senior doctor, such as a consultant, or specialist or specialty registrar. This assessor grades your performance, completes the observation tool, and provides you with feedback. The completed report is kept in your portfolio, as evidence of competence.

2. Case-based discussion (CBD)

A CBD is a structured review of a case of your choosing, but it must be one in which you were professionally involved. It involves a discussion with a senior doctor, usually a consultant, of your decision-making and clinical reasoning in that particular case. Again, the assessor grades your performance and provides feedback.

3. Multi-source feedback

This is similar to a 360 degree assessment, and involves you asking your colleagues to rate your abilities and to offer comments on different aspects of your work as a doctor, including performance, clinical ability, attitudes, and professionalism. The three tools currently in use are:

- the Mini Peer Assessment Tool (mini-PAT)
- Team Assessment of Behaviours (TAB)
- a multi-source feedback tool (in Scotland).

You have to identify colleagues from a variety of different disciplines to act as assessors and to complete these assessments for you. The process of completing the assessments will vary locally. However, the process is meant to be anonymous; only the results of a compiled report, which is sent to your educational supervisor, will be available to you. A report will be generated only when a minimum required number of assessments have been submitted, so you should choose your assessors wisely.

2 A guide to the UK Foundation schools

Mark J Portou

The aim of this chapter is to consolidate the pertinent aspects of the available information regarding each of the Foundation schools in the UK into one convenient location. You can then refer to this material before you submit an application. For each of the Foundation schools, information regarding its geographical location, the major hospital trusts within the Foundation school, contact details and web addresses are provided as a minimum. In addition, further details are included for some Foundation schools where available. It should be noted, however, that this information, and indeed the lists within this chapter, are not meant to be exhaustive. Further, the amount of information provided for each Foundation school merely reflects that available in the public domain, and you should not try to use it as a means to differentiate between Foundation schools.

The detail of this chapter does not reflect personal opinion. Rather, the intention is to present the information in an unbiased and objective way. Ultimately, the decision regarding choice of Foundation school is of course left entirely to you.

Further detailed information regarding each of the Foundation schools can be found on the website of the Foundation Programme, at www.foundationprogramme.nhs.uk/pages/home/deaneries-foundation-schools.

Foundation schools

Foundation schools are the educational bodies that oversee the delivery of Foundation training across the country. They comprise medical schools, the local educational deanery, individual hospital trusts, primary care trusts (PCTs), and other establishments (e.g. hospices) that offer Foundation doctors training in a range of different settings and clinical environments. The Foundation schools also orchestrate the formal teaching programmes and provide local guidance on the national Foundation Programme assessment framework.

There are presently (since the merger of South East Thames and South West Thames) 26 Foundation schools nationwide. Their capacity is indicated in Table 2.1.

Foundation schools: an applicant's guide

It is crucial that you choose a Foundation school that satisfies your individual needs. Historically, most doctors have elected to stay in the familiar environment of the medical school in which they trained. However, with the advent of a centralized, anonymous, national application system, there is no longer a home advantage. Thus, you must consider and thoroughly research your choice of Foundation school, and take into account not just the rotations and programmes on offer across the 2 years, but also the reputation of the Foundation school and the region of the country. It is useful to visit the Foundation school and individual trust websites, and, even better, to visit the area in person, before you make your application. After all, 2 years is a long time to live with a poor choice.

Birmingham North Foundation School
http://wmsha.com

The Foundation Programme is run out of City Hospital, Sandwell Hospital, Good Hope Hospital, Heartlands Hospital, and Solihull Hospital. These trusts cover the diverse populations of the northern, central, and eastern parts of the city, which include both

Table 2.1 Numbers of Foundation school vacancies and local students, 2007. Adapted from www.foundationprogramme.nhs.uk.

	Vacancies	Local students
Birmingham North	111	567[a]
Birmingham South	111	567[a]
Black Country	7	567[a]
Coventry and Warwick	85	567[a]
East Anglian	147	137
Hereford and Worcestershire	66	567[a]
Keele	155	567[a]
Leicestershire, Northamptonshire and Rutland	130	223
Mersey	266	284
North Central Thames	306	381
North East Thames	264	303
North West Thames	306	361
North Western	485	406
North Yorkshire and East Coast	157	292[b]
Northern Deanery	348	322
Northern Ireland	210	193
Oxford	168	140
Peninsula	148	92
Scottish	803	846
Severn	246	194
South East Thames[c]	381	384
South West Thames[c]	279	265
South Yorkshire	156	259
Trent	270	321
Wales	312	302
Wessex	217	186
West Yorkshire	250	292[b]

[a] Total for West Midlands as a whole.
[b] Total for Yorkshire as a whole.
[c] Now combined as South Thames.

densely populated inner-city areas and some more affluent suburbs. The school states that:

- 'It is committed to receiving and acting on trainee feedback. All teaching programmes are carefully evaluated and are regularly updated both in style and in content.'
- 'It has well established careers support programmes and pastoral care schemes.'
- 'It offers experienced Clinical Tutors, diverse placement opportunities including Paediatrics at the Birmingham Children's Hospital, Public Health, Genito-Urinary Medicine, Infectious Diseases Medicine, Critical Care, Accident & Emergency in both Foundation year 1 (F1) and 2 (F2), Dermatology and Laboratory Medicine. In F2 there are large numbers of GP placements available and the University of Birmingham recognised Postgraduate Award in Generic Skills.'

Hospital trusts

Heart of England NHS Foundation Trust
Sandwell and West Birmingham NHS Trust

Contact

St Chad's Court, 213 Hagley Road, Edgbaston, Birmingham B16 9RG
Tel: 0845 155 1022

Birmingham South Foundation School

http://wmsha.com

The Birmingham South Foundation School has 'a lively and dynamic training programme offering unique experience in general and specialist trusts providing acute hospital and community based services in primary, secondary and tertiary care'. The objective of all the Birmingham South programmes is to develop a sound foundation for entry into future specialty training.

Hospital trusts

Birmingham Children's Hospital Foundation NHS Trust

Birmingham and Solihull Mental Health Trust
University Hospitals Birmingham Foundation NHS Trust

Contact

St Chad's Court, 213 Hagley Road, Edgbaston,
Birmingham B16 9RG
Tel: 0845 155 1022

Black Country Foundation School
http://wmsha.com

The Black Country Foundation School covers the geographical
area to the west of Birmingham. Wolverhampton, Dudley, and
Walsall, along with West Bromwich, make up the Black Country;
all have large, diverse, urban populations.

Hospital trusts

Dudley Group of Hospitals NHS Trust
Royal Wolverhampton Hospitals NHS Trust
Walsall Hospitals NHS Trust

Contact

St Chad's Court, 213 Hagley Road, Edgbaston,
Birmingham B16 9RG
Tel: 0845 155 1022

Coventry and Warwick Foundation School
http://wmsha.com

The Coventry and Warwick Foundation School offers 2-year
Foundation Programmes based around University Hospital in
Coventry, George Eliot Hospital in Nuneaton, and South
Warwickshire Hospital in Warwick. Most rotations at F1 are
across two trusts, and all include general surgery and acute
medicine as 4-month placements. All F2 rotations have acute
medicine in some form (including accident and emergency, and

intensive care medicine), and a wide range of other specialties. The teaching programme at F1 occurs in modern educational facilities at the three trusts and is based on a common curriculum across the school. At F2, trainees come together for one afternoon a week at University Hospital in the large modern Clinical Science Building.

The school states that: 'all foundation trainees have a portfolio-based online learning log, which documents their experience and progress over the two years. The assessment programme is comprehensive; application for a particular F2 rotation is based on preferences and performance at F1. All F2 doctors, as part of their generic skills training, will enrol for a Postgraduate Award (PGA) in Professional Skills at Warwick University.'

Hospital trusts

George Eliot Hospital NHS Trust
South Warwickshire General Hospitals NHS Trust
University Hospitals Coventry and Warwickshire NHS Trust

Contact

St Chad's Court, 213 Hagley Road, Edgbaston, Birmingham B16 9RG
Tel: 0845 155 1022

East Anglian Foundation School

www.easterndeanery.org

The East Anglian Foundation School covers a large area in the east of England, including the counties of Cambridgeshire, Norfolk, Suffolk, Bedfordshire, and Hertfordshire.

Hospital trusts

Bedford Hospital NHS Trust
Cambridge University Hospitals NHS Foundation Trust
East and North Hertfordshire NHS Trust
Hinchingbrooke Health Care NHS Trust

Ipswich Hospital NHS Trust
James Paget University Hospitals NHS Foundation Trust
Luton and Dunstable Hospital NHS Foundation Trust
Norfolk and Norwich University Hospitals NHS Foundation Trust
Papworth Hospital NHS Foundation Trust
Peterborough and Stamford Hospitals NHS Foundation Trust
Queen Elizabeth Hospital, King's Lynn, NHS Trust
West Suffolk Hospital NHS Trust

Contact

East of England Deanery, Block 3, Ida Darwin,
Fulbourn, Cambridge CB21 5EE
Email: foundationprogramme.enquiries@eoe.nhs.uk
Tel: 01223 884848

Hereford and Worcestershire Foundation School
http://wmsha.com

The Hereford and Worcestershire Foundation School is located in the southernmost region of the West Midlands deanery. It covers the rural counties of Herefordshire and Worcestershire.

Hospital trusts

Herefordshire Hospitals NHS Trust
Worcestershire Acute Hospitals NHS Trust

Contact

St Chad's Court, 213 Hagley Road, Edgbaston,
Birmingham B16 9RG
Tel: 0845 155 1022

Keele Foundation School
http://wmsha.com

This Foundation School is found to the north of the West Midlands, in the counties of Shropshire and Staffordshire.

Hospital trusts

> Burton Hospital NHS Trust
> Mid-Staffordshire Hospital NHS Trust
> Shrewsbury and Telford NHS Trust
> University Hospital of North Staffordshire NHS Trust

Contact

> St Chad's Court, 213 Hagley Road, Edgbaston,
> Birmingham B16 9RG
> Tel: 0845 155 1022

Leicestershire, Northamptonshire and Rutland Foundation School

www.eastmidlandsdeanery.nhs.uk

> In Leicestershire, Northamptonshire and Rutland (LNR), F1 will consist of three 4-month placements. All F1 trainees at the University Hospitals of Leicester receive a copy of the Foundation learning portfolio, which aims to guide trainees through Foundation Programme learning and provides a record of progress through the Foundation Programme. F1 doctors appointed to 2-year programmes may use up to 5 days of their F2 study leave allocation for a clinical (taster) attachment. LNR supports The Royal College of Surgeons of England Affiliates' membership scheme.

Hospital trusts

> Kettering General Hospital NHS Trust
> Leicestershire Partnership NHS Trust
> Northampton General Hospital NHS Trust
> University Hospitals of Leicester NHS Trust

Contact

> Foundation School Office, 11 Merus Court,
> Meridian Business Park, Leicester LE19 1RJ
> Tel: 0115 846 7125

Mersey Foundation School
www.merseydeanery.nhs.uk

A 1-year generic training programme, support in developing a learning portfolio, and regular educational appraisal with a consultant educator are available in all F1 placements. These placements are intended to provide individuals with the generic and acute care skills to be able to identify and manage the acutely ill patient.

Hospital trusts

Aintree University Hospitals NHS Foundation Trust
Countess of Chester NHS Foundation Trust
East Cheshire NHS Trust
Mid-Cheshire Hospitals NHS Trust
North Cheshire Hospitals NHS Trust
Royal Liverpool and Broadgreen University Hospitals NHS Trust
Southport and Ormskirk Hospitals NHS Trust
St Helens and Knowsley NHS Trust
Wirral Hospitals NHS Trust

Contact

Mersey Deanery, Regatta Place, Brunswick Business Park,
Summers Road, Liverpool L3 4BL
Tel: 0151 285 4700/4701

North Central Thames Foundation School
www.ucl.ac.uk/medicalschool/nctfs

The North Central Thames Foundation School (NCTFS) is a school of the London Deanery, based at The Royal Free and University College Medical School (RFUCMS). NCTFS has training programmes in six London Deanery trusts and five Eastern Deanery trusts. These extend to Basildon and Southend in the east, and Luton and Stevenage in the north. The Foundation school coordinates the allocation processes to F1 and F2, and supports the delivery of Foundation training and the development of trainees.

London Deanery hospital trusts

Barking, Havering Redbridge Hospitals NHS Trust
Barnet and Chase Farm Hospitals NHS Trust
North Middlesex University Hospital NHS Trust
Royal Free Hampstead NHS Trust
University College London Hospitals NHS Foundation Trust
Whittington Hospital NHS Trust

Eastern Deanery hospital trusts

Basildon and Thurrock University NHS Foundation Trust
East and North Hertfordshire NHS Trust
Luton and Dunstable Hospital NHS Foundation Trust
Princess Alexandra Hospital NHS Trust
Southend University Hospital NHS Foundation Trust
West Hertfordshire Hospitals NHS Trust

Contact

North Central Thames Foundation School, Royal Free and University College Medical School, Rowland Hill Street, London NW3 2PF
Email: nctfs@medsch.ucl.ac.uk
Tel: 020 7472 6555

North East Thames Foundation School

www.netfs.org.uk

North East Thames Foundation School was established by the London Deanery in collaboration with Barts and The London School of Medicine and Dentistry and the East of England Deanery. Foundation Programme training (F1 and F2) is designed to give Foundation doctors a range of experience before they choose an area of medicine in which to specialize and delivers an integrated educational programme with defined outcomes.

Hospital trusts

> Barking, Havering Redbridge Hospitals NHS Trust
> Barts and The London NHS Trust (BLT)
> East London NHS Foundation Trust
> Homerton University Hospital NHS Foundation Trust
> Newham University Hospital NHS Trust
> North East London Mental Health NHS Trust
> Whipps Cross University Hospital NHS Trust

Contact

> North East Thames Foundation School, 31–43 Ashfield Street,
> London E1 2AH
> Email: enquiries@netfs.org.uk

North West Thames Foundation School

www1.imperial.ac.uk/medicine/teaching/prho

> The North West Thames Foundation School is a partnership
> between Imperial College London and the London Deanery; it
> incorporates Foundation training programmes within linked
> NHS trusts and deaneries, covering a wide geographical area.

Hospital trusts

> Chelsea and Westminster NHS Foundation Trust
> Ealing Hospital NHS Trust
> Essex Rivers Healthcare NHS Trust
> Hillingdon Hospital NHS Trust
> Imperial College Healthcare NHS Trust
> North West London Hospitals NHS Trust
> West Hertfordshire Hospitals NHS Trust
> West Middlesex University Hospital NHS Trust

Contact

> Email: umo-nwtfs@imperial.ac.uk
> Tel: 020 7589 5111

North Western Foundation School
www.nwpgmd.nhs.uk

The North Western Deanery incorporates the counties of Greater Manchester, Lancashire and Cumbria.

Hospital trusts

Blackpool, Fylde and Wyre NHS Trust
Bolton Hospitals NHS Trust
Central Manchester and Manchester Children's University Trust
East Lancashire Hospitals NHS Trust
Pennine Acute Hospitals NHS Trust
Salford Royal Hospitals NHS Trust
Stockport NHS Foundation Trust
Trafford Healthcare NHS Trust
University Hospitals of Morecombe Bay NHS Trust
Wrightington, Wigan and Leigh NHS Trust

Contact

North Western Deanery, 4th Floor, Barlow House,
Minshull Street, Manchester M1 3DZ
Tel: 0161 237 3690

North Yorkshire and East Coast Foundation School
www.nyecpgme.org.uk

The North Yorkshire and East Coast Foundation School (NYEC) started in August 2005. An additional 37 F1 programmes were added in August 2007, with a proportionate increase in F2 numbers. This expansion was expected to continue again in August 2008, when the first Hull York Medical School graduates were due to enter F1. All trainees spend each year in a different trust, with 1 year in a teaching hospital and 1 year in a district general hospital. All F1 programmes include general medicine and general surgery. All F2 programmes aspire to provide one primary care post and one acute care post. F2 programmes are selected by trainees from a list of complementary programmes, through a collaborative matching process, with no scores, no forms, and no interviews. All trainees attend a mandatory generic skills programme tailored to meet the requirements of the Foundation curriculum.

Hospital trusts

Hull and East Yorkshire Hospitals NHS Trust
Northern Lincolnshire and Goole Hospitals NHS Trust
Scarborough and North East Yorkshire NHS Trust
York Hospitals NHS Foundation Trust

Contact

NYEC Foundation School, Hertford Building, University of Hull, Cottingham Road, Hull HU6 7RX
Email: manager@foundation.nyecpgme.org.uk
Tel: 01482 463400

Northern Deanery Foundation School
http://mypimd.ncl.ac.uk

The Northern Deanery Foundation School (NDFS) states that it aims to support the 'delivery of excellence in healthcare in the North East through ensuring excellence in FP [Foundation Programme] Training'. Foundation training has been successfully established within the NDFS, which works in partnership with the nine acute trusts in the region. The Foundation Programme team works with a wide variety of organizations and colleagues, mainly Newcastle University, NHS trusts, strategic health authorities, regional GP networks, the Department of Health, the GMC, and the Postgraduate Medical Education and Training Board (PMETB).

Hospital trusts

City Hospitals Sunderland NHS Foundation Trust
County Durham and Darlington NHS Foundation Trust
Gateshead Health NHS Foundation Trust
Newcastle upon Tyne Hospitals NHS Foundation Trust
North Cumbria Acute Hospitals NHS Trust

North Tees and Hartlepool Acute NHS Trust
Northumbria Healthcare NHS Foundation Trust
South Tees Hospitals NHS Trust
South Tyneside NHS Foundation Trust

Contact

Northern Deanery, 10–12 Framlington Place,
Newcastle upon Tyne NE2 4AB
Email: ndfsinfo@cddft.nhs.uk
Tel: 0191 222 8923

Northern Ireland Foundation School

www.nimdta.gov.uk

There are 14 Foundation Programmes in Northern Ireland. The Foundation Programme director ensures that trainees' regular appraisals take place and that learning and development portfolios are supported within the process, as well as offering career advice and ensuring that individual trainees receive the necessary training to gain the competences required. An educational supervisor is responsible for a group of up to 15 trainees, and ensures that the assessment takes place; supervisors also decide whether individual placements have been completed. A clinical supervisor is responsible for teaching and supervising Foundation trainees and conducting assessments.

Hospital trusts

Altnagelvin Area Hospital Trust
Belfast City Hospital Trust
Causeway Trust
Craigavon Area Hospital Trust
Down Lisburn Trust
Foyle Trust
Royal Group of Hospitals Trust
Sperrin Lakeland Trust
Ulster Hospitals Trust
United Hospitals Trust

Contact

NIMDTA, Beechill House, 42 Beechill Road, Belfast BT8 7RL
Email: foundation@nimdta.gov.uk
Tel: 028 9040 0000

Oxford Foundation School

www.oxford-pgmde.co.uk

The Oxford Foundation School is located in the counties of Oxfordshire, Buckinghamshire, and Berkshire. It was anticipated that 228 posts would be available in 2008, although this figure, including the post content, is provisional and subject to change.

Hospital trusts

Buckinghamshire Hospitals NHS Trust
Heatherwood and Wexham Park Hospitals NHS Trust
Milton Keynes Hospital NHS Foundation Trust
Oxford Radcliffe Hospitals NHS Trust
Royal Berkshire NHS Foundation Trust

Contact

The Triangle, Roosevelt Drive, Headington, Oxford OX3 7XP
Email: modmedcar@oxford-pgmde.co.uk
Tel: 01865 740601

Peninsula Foundation School

www.pms.ac.uk/peninsuladeanery_cms

The Peninsula Foundation School covers the counties of Devon and Cornwall, in the south-west of England. The School operates under the control of the South West Peninsula Deanery and exists to ensure that the educational infrastructure required to deliver a high-quality Foundation Programme is in place.

BARTS & THE LONDON SMD

Hospital trusts

Northern Devon Healthcare NHS Trust
Plymouth Hospitals NHS Trust
Royal Cornwall Hospitals NHS Trust
Royal Devon and Exeter Foundation Trust
South Devon Healthcare NHS Trust

Contact

The John Bull Building, Tamar Science Park, Plymouth PL6 8BU
Email: F1enquiries@peninsuladeanery.ac.uk
01752 437436

Scottish Foundation School

www.nes.scot.nhs.uk/medicine/foundation

The Scottish Foundation School covers the whole of Scotland. It encompasses the four Scottish Deaneries – North, South-East, East, and West – which are part of NHS Education for Scotland. The School provides a wide range of programmes, covering different types of population, at remote and rural hospitals as well as teaching hospitals, and many specialties. In addition, it also provides a number of academic programmes.

East Region

Ninewells Hospital and Medical School, Dundee
Perth Royal Infirmary
Stracathro Hospital, Brechin

South-East Region

Borders General Hospital, Melrose
Queen Margaret Hospital, Dunfermline
Royal Hospital for Sick Children, Edinburgh
Royal Infirmary of Edinburgh
St John's Hospital, Livingston
Victoria Hospital, Kirkcaldy
Western General Hospital

North Region

Aberdeen Maternity Hospital
Aberdeen Royal Infirmary
Balfour Hospital, Kirkwall
Belford Hospital, Fort William
Caithness General Hospital, Wick
Dr Gray's Hospital, Elgin
Gilbert Bain Hospital, Lerwick
New Craig's Hospital, Inverness
Raigmore Hospital, Inverness
Roxburghe House, Aberdeen
Royal Aberdeen Children's Hospital
Royal Cornhill Hospital, Aberdeen
Western Isles Hospital
Woodend Hospital, Aberdeen

West Region

Ayr Hospital
Crosshouse Hospital, Kilmarnock
Dumfries and Galloway Royal Infirmary
Falkirk Royal Infirmary
Gartnavel General Hospital
Glasgow Royal Infirmary
Hairmyres Hospital
Inverclyde Royal Hospital, Greenock
Lorn and Islands District General Hospital, Oban
Monklands Hospital, Airdrie
Royal Alexandra Hospital, Paisley
Royal Hospital for Sick Children
Southern General Hospital
Stirling Royal Infirmary
Stobhill Hospital
Vale of Leven District General Hospital
Victoria Infirmary
Western Infirmary
Wishaw General Hospital

East Region contact

Postgraduate Medical Office (Level 7), Ninewells Hospital and
Medical School, Dundee DD1 9SY

North Region contact

> Forest Grove House, Foresterhill Road, Aberdeen AB25 2ZP
> Tel: 01224 554365

South-East Region contact

> The Lister, 11 Hill Square, Edinburgh EH8 9DR
> Tel: 0131 650 2609

West Region contact

> 3rd Floor, 2 Central Quay, 89 Hydepark Street, Glasgow G3 8BW
> Tel: 0141 223 1400/1401

Severn Foundation School

www.severndeanery.nhs.uk/severn_foundation_school.shtml

> The Severn Foundation School is situated in the west of England, and incorporates the counties of Gloucestershire, Wiltshire, Somerset, and Devon.

Hospital trusts

> Gloucestershire Hospitals NHS Foundation Trust
> North Bristol NHS Trust
> Northern Devon Healthcare NHS Trust
> Royal United Hospital Bath NHS Trust
> South Devon Healthcare NHS Trust
> Swindon & Marlborough NHS Trust
> Taunton & Somerset NHS Trust
> United Bristol Healthcare NHS Trust
> Weston Area Health NHS Trust
> Yeovil District Hospital NHS Foundation Trust

Contact

> Severn Deanery, Academic Centre, Frenchay Hospital,
> Bristol BS16 1LE
> Email: clare.moorcroft@southwest.nhs.uk
> Tel: 0117 975 7033

South Thames Foundation School
www.stfs.org.uk

A single South Thames Foundation School was formed in October 2007 following the merger of the former Brighton, South East Thames, and South West Thames Foundation Schools. The South Thames Foundation School has been established in collaboration with the Kent, Surrey and Sussex (KSS) and London Postgraduate Deaneries, and King's College, London, St George's University of London, and Brighton and Sussex Medical Schools. It manages all F1 and F2 trainees (approximately 1700) in NHS trusts in the South London and KSS regions and is based in three offices, at London Bridge, and in Brighton and Tooting.

Hospital trusts

Brighton and Sussex University Hospitals NHS Trust
Bromley Hospitals NHS Trust
Dartford and Gravesham NHS Trust
East Kent Hospitals NHS Trust
East Somerset NHS Trust
East Sussex Hospitals NHS Trust
Epsom and St Helier University Hospitals NHS Trust
Frimley Park Hospital NHS Foundation Trust
Guy's and St Thomas' NHS Foundation Trust
Isle of Wight Healthcare NHS Trust
Jersey NHS Trust
King's College Hospital NHS Trust
Kingston Hospital NHS Trust
Lewisham Hospital NHS Trust
Maidstone and Tunbridge Wells Hospitals NHS Trust
Mayday Healthcare NHS Trust
Medway Hospital NHS Trust
North Hampshire Hospitals NHS Trust
Northern Devon Healthcare NHS Trust
Plymouth Hospitals NHS Trust
Queen Elizabeth Hospital NHS Trust
Queen Mary's Sidcup NHS Trust
Royal Surrey County Hospital NHS Trust
Royal West Sussex NHS Trust
St George's Healthcare NHS Trust

Surrey and Sussex Healthcare NHS Trust
Worthing and Southlands Hospitals NHS Trust

Contact

Sherman Education Centre, 4th Floor, Southwark Wing, Guy's Hospital, Great Maze Pond, London SE1 9RT
Email: enquiries@stfs.org.uk
Tel: 020 7188 9591

South Yorkshire Foundation School

www.syshdeanery.com

The South Yorkshire Foundation School was established in collaboration with the South Yorkshire and South Humber Postgraduate Deanery and the University of Sheffield. It manages all F1 and F2 trainees in NHS trusts in Sheffield, Rotherham, Barnsley, Chesterfield, Doncaster, and Bassetlaw, and is based at Don Valley House in Sheffield.

Hospital trusts

Barnsley Hospital NHS Foundation Trust
Chesterfield Royal Hospital NHS Foundation Trust
Doncaster and Bassetlaw Hospitals NHS Foundation Hospitals
Rotherham District General Hospital NHS Trust
Sheffield Care Trust
Sheffield Children's NHS Foundation Trust
Sheffield Teaching Hospitals NHS Foundation Trust

Contact

Don Valley House, Saville Street East, Sheffield S4 7UQ
Email: sarah.chown@yorksandhumber.nhs.uk
Tel: 0114 226 4451

Trent Foundation School

www.eastmidlandsdeanery.nhs.uk

The Trent Foundation School covers a wide area from the Derbyshire–Staffordshire border on the west to the North Sea on the Lincolnshire coastline. The area is diverse, consisting of both industrial and rural areas. The Foundation School is one of two within the East Midlands Healthcare Workforce Deanery and covers the areas of Derbyshire, Nottinghamshire, and the majority of Lincolnshire, excluding the area along the River Humber corridor. Foundation trainees are sent to five acute trusts, a number of which have more than one hospital in them.

Hospital trusts

Chesterfield Royal Hospital NHS Foundation Trust
Derby Hospitals NHS Foundation Trust
Lincoln County Hospital, Lincoln
Louth Hospital, Lincolnshire
Nottingham University Hospitals NHS Trust
Pilgrim Hospital, Boston, Lincolnshire
Sherwood Forest Hospitals NHS Foundation Trust
United Lincolnshire Hospitals NHS Foundation Trust

Contact

East Midlands Healthcare Workforce Deanery, Kings Meadow Campus, Lenton Lane, University of Nottingham, Nottingham NG7 2NA
Email: Heidi.Breed@nottingham.ac.uk
Tel: 0115 846 7121

Wales Foundation School

www.mmcwales.org/foundation-programmes

Hospital trusts

Bro Morgannwg NHS Trust
Cardiff and Vale NHS Trust
Carmarthenshire NHS Trust

Ceredigion and Mid Wales NHS Trust
Conwy and Denbighshire NHS Trust
Gwent Healthcare NHS Trust
North East Wales NHS Trust
North Glamorgan NHS Trust
North West Wales NHS Trust
Pembrokeshire and Derwen NHS Trust
Pontypridd and Rhondda NHS Trust
Swansea NHS Trust

Contact

School of Postgraduate Medical & Dental Education, Cardiff University, Neuadd Meirionnydd, Heath Park, Cardiff CF14 4XN
Email: daviesje8@cardiff.ac.uk
Tel: 029 2068 7455

Wessex Foundation School

www.nesc.nhs.uk

The Wessex Foundation School is located in the south of England, and covers the counties of Hampshire, Dorset, Isle of Wight, Wiltshire, and Jersey.

Hospital trusts

Basingstoke and North Hampshire NHS Foundation Trust
Dorset County Hospital NHS Foundation Trust
Isle of Wight Healthcare NHS Trust
Jersey General Hospital Trust
Poole Hospital NHS Foundation Trust
Portsmouth Hospitals NHS Trust
Ridgeway Partnership
Royal Bournemouth and Christchurch NHS Foundation Trust
Salisbury NHS Foundation Trust
Southampton University Hospitals NHS Trust
Winchester and Eastleigh Healthcare NHS Trust

Contact

Email: wessexfs.enquiries@nesc.nhs.uk

West Yorkshire Foundation School
www.wyfs.nhs.uk

The West Yorkshire Foundation School is located in the central north of England, and incorporates NHS organizations from Airdale, Bradford, Calderdale, Harrogate, Huddersfield, Leeds, Pontefract, and Wakefield.

Hospital trusts

Airedale NHS Trust
Bradford Teaching Hospitals NHS Trust
Calderdale and Huddersfield NHS Trust
Harrogate and District NHS Foundation Trust
Leeds Teaching Hospitals NHS Trust
Mid-Yorkshire Hospitals NHS Trust

Contact

Email: wyfsenquiries@nhs.net

3 The application process for the Foundation Programme

Mark J Portou, Manoj Ramachandran, and Marc A Gladman

Applications for Foundation training

All applications for entry to the Foundation Programme in every Foundation school in England, Scotland, Wales, and Northern Ireland are made via a centralized, secure website, www.foundationprogramme.nhs.uk.

The application process runs to a national timetable, outside of which it is impossible to submit an application. The website, however, remains open and provides links to the individual Foundation schools' websites, and lists some general information on the process, as well as frequently asked questions (FAQs); it is also due to have a users' forum. Also included is a downloadable Foundation applicant's handbook, which provides some basic guidance on how to approach the individual questions.

For 2008 entry, the process took place over a 12-day period between 29 October and 9 November 2007. Only during this time were applicants actually able to submit completed forms onto the website. Any applicant attempting to submit an application after 9 November would find the relevant task bar missing from the website and thus miss out.

Long before the application form is ever seen, guidance is published on which candidates are suitable for acceptance on the Foundation Programme. The 'eligibility criteria' and 'person specification' (see below) were in fact available on the website on 8 August 2007.

Registering

Before you can make an application, you must first register at www.foundationprogramme.nhs.uk. This can be done once the application process has opened. Registering is fairly easy; it requires you to visit the website and click on 'register and enrol'. The onscreen instructions tell you to select a login and password. An authentication code is then emailed to you.

Eligibility criteria

The eligibility criteria can be found in a two-page document available for download (under the 'Faculty' tab's 'Application process' page). They define those persons who are entitled to apply to the UK Foundation Programme. Doctors who have achieved full GMC registration, or who are eligible for it by virtue of their previous experience, are excluded from applications to the full 2-year Foundation Programme. The exceptions to this rule are overseas doctors who have full registration but who have not yet completed an internship in a UK hospital.

The eligibility criteria as published for 2008 entry were as follows:

1. Applicants must have the written approval of their medical school's dean (or equivalent) to apply. Any applicants from a UK medical school will have this done on their behalf after successfully completing their undergraduate training, and subsequently qualifying.
2. Applicants must have a verifiable academic rating determined by their medical school, as set out in a statement by the dean (or equivalent) of the applicant's medical school. This is essentially the applicant's academic position in the medical school year, listed like a league table. In addition, applicants from outside the UK must provide transcripts in English of all undergraduate grades.
3. Applicants must have a valid medical degree, recognized by the GMC for UK professional medical registration, and have obtained provisional registration with the GMC, and be in a

position to take up a post (exact start date to be agreed with the employer). This requirement means that those international medical graduate (IMG) applicants who require successful completion of the PLAB (Professional and Linguistic Assessment Board) test, in order to allow sufficient time to obtain GMC registration; they will, of course, also have to meet, and provide appropriate evidence for, all the other relevant GMC criteria. Obviously, all graduates from UK medical schools will have recognized degrees. The term 'international medical graduates' (IMGs) refers to doctors who are not born in the UK or European Union, and who did not graduate from a medical school in the UK, and are thus required by the GMC to complete the PLAB examination.

4. Applicants must have the right to work in the UK, or be a student of a UK medical school in their final year of study with existing leave as a student. Applicants who require a work permit to take up employment may be considered only if there are insufficient suitable applicants who do not require a work permit. This will automatically include those with British and European Union passports/nationality.

5. Applicants must be available to take up their Foundation Programme. All new Foundation Programme jobs nationwide start in the first week in August.

6. Applicants must be fit to practise medicine safely, in accordance with the GMC document *Good Medical Practice* (2006) (available for download from www.gmc-uk.org).

7. Applicants must have sufficient skill in written and spoken English to enable effective communication about medical topics with patients and colleagues. This could be demonstrated by either applicants having undertaken their entire undergraduate medical training in English or applicants having attained the minimum International English Language Testing System (IELTS) score (minimum scores: overall 7.5, speaking 7.5, listening 7.5, reading 7.5, writing 7.5). The Eligibility Office reserves the right to verify English language skills through the use of telephone assessments if there is some doubt about the standard of the English language skills demonstrated in the application. In addition, face-to-face interviews may be required to assess these skills.

8. Applicants must have graduated from medical school within 2 years of commencement of the 2008 Foundation Programme, that is, on or after 31 July 2006. If graduation was more than 2 years earlier, applicants must provide evidence of maintaining clinical knowledge and skills. Applicants in the latter category may need to undergo an assessment to ensure that their clinical knowledge and skills have been maintained to the extent that they are appropriate for entry to the Foundation Programme.
9. Applicants must provide references in the manner set out in the application guidance.

For British graduates and those from within the European Union, the evidence required to confirm eligibility is provided by the applicant's medical school.

Person specification

The person specification describes the minimum requirements expected of successful Foundation Programme applicants. It is also available for download (again, under the 'Faculty' tab's 'Application process' page). It is divided into six categories:

- eligibility
- qualifications
- clinical knowledge and skills
- language skills
- personal skills
- probity.

For each category, specific examples of how the applicant should meet these criteria are given in a table, which has a third column outlining how these criteria will be assessed in the application process. The vast majority of these skills will be assessed from the application form alone, in the eligibility sections, personal sections, and, of course, the questions. If there is any doubt of the applicant's ability to meet these person specifications, a telephone interview may, in some circumstances, be necessary.

The person specifications for entry to the Foundation Programme can be found in the Appendix to this book.

The application form

The online complete form is released several weeks before the application process opens, which gives you plenty of time to become familiar with it. The application form is divided into several different sections, as follows.

Personal details

The first part of the application form is very simple. You need only give your name, address, and telephone number.

Other information

This section takes the form of a drop-down menu (yes/no) and a blank box. In the event of a 'yes' answer for any of these questions, you are required to give details in free text in the box.

It is important to mention that the scorers of the application form will not have access to the answers of this section of the form, and therefore the answers that you give here cannot affect your score. (The scoring process is described in detail in Chapter 4.)

Disability Discrimination Act

This blank space offers you the opportunity to declare any disabilities, under the Disabilities Discrimination Act 1995. If you do not consider that you have a disability, you can leave this blank.

Rehabilitation of Offenders Act ('spent' and 'unspent' convictions)

As set out in the Rehabilitation of Offenders Act 1974, applicants for most jobs are *not* required to disclose previous convictions to potential employers after they have served a rehabilitation period, which is set by the courts on conviction. If the applicant has not yet completed this rehabilitation period, it is referred to as an 'unspent' conviction and must be disclosed. Medical jobs are exempt from the Rehabilitation of Offenders Act, however, owing to their public service nature and access to sensitive information; therefore, even convictions, cautions, and warnings that are 'spent' *must* be disclosed, and a box is provided for this purpose.

Relationships

This is where you must declare whether you have a relationship with a director or other employee of the appointing organization, which might highlight a major conflict of interest.

Fitness to practise

This asks whether your fitness to practise has been called into doubt, by ascertaining whether you are under any investigation or disciplinary proceedings by any regulatory body, which in the UK is, of course, the GMC. If so, the question requires you to give the details surrounding this investigation, including the reason and the exact restrictions placed on your practice by the regulatory body.

Qualifications

GMC registration

As indicated above, the eligibility criteria state that Foundation Programme doctors should be pre-registration with the GMC; you will probably, therefore, select 'I do not have GMC registration' from the drop-down menu. The exceptions to this are also available in this menu.

Main medical degree

This asks for the medical degree that you are undertaking (e.g. MBBS, MBChB), the date that you entered medical school, and the school's name and address. The vast majority of applicants will be applying from medical school, and thus will have to give an expected rather than an actual date of qualification.

Post-qualification

This applies only to applicants who have already qualified, and who have already worked as a doctor. This box allows them to record that postgraduate experience, but it will be left blank in the case of those applying from medical school.

Other educational qualifications

In this section, up to four additional qualifications may be mentioned. Only recognized qualifications are suitable for listing here. Degrees such as an intercalated BSc, MSc, or PhD should be mentioned.

Clinical and practical skills training and experience

The clinical and practical skills section of the form requires a certain amount of self-reflection. A number of clinical skills are listed that have been identified by the GMC as being particularly important for medical graduates. You are required to self-certify your competence in these skills, by selecting the yes or no options for each. The scorers of the form (see Chapter 4) will not see this self-certified list, but it will be passed on to your future employing trust once the selection process is complete, and you are, therefore, urged to be honest, if only to allow for extra training in order to gain these competences.

The clinical skills listed on previous application forms were:

- Take and record a patient's history, including the family history.
- Perform a full physical examination and a mental state examination.
- Interpret the findings from the history, the physical examination, and the mental state examination.
- Interpret the results of commonly used investigations.
- Make clinical decisions based on the gathered evidence.
- Assess a patient's problems and form plans to investigate and manage these, involving patients in the planning process.

- Work out drug dosage and record the outcome accurately.
- Write safe prescriptions for different types of drugs.
- Perform venepuncture.
- Insert a cannula into peripheral veins.
- Give intravenous injections.
- Give intramuscular and subcutaneous injections.
- Carry out arterial blood sampling.
- Perform suturing.
- Demonstrate competency in basic life support.
- Carry out basic respiratory function tests.
- Administer oxygen therapy.
- Use a nebulizer correctly.
- Nasogastric tube insertion.
- Perform bladder catheterization.

'White space' answers

The fields discussed above are all mandatory, that is, they must be completed to allow the form to be successfully submitted, and enable identification of those who are eligible to apply. However, they do not carry any points. The remainder of the form is where you pick up scores for your application. The application form questions are in the form of 'white space' (free text) answers.

The 'white space' questions set out to test whether you have the key attributes required of a Foundation doctor, as set out in the person specification. Knowledge of this document is pivotal when answering the questions. Each question examines a different attribute, such as identification of the patient as the central focus of care, or the ability to communicate with colleagues and patients. Most questions ask for an example, and for evidence of learning and reflection, while specifically addressing the relevance to Foundation training. These questions are the focus of Chapters 5–11.

Major question themes

From year to year, the exact wording of the individual questions is likely to change. This is not surprising, as each year's application form must be different enough to prevent obvious resubmission of successful answers from previous applicants, and thus prevent plagiarism.

There are, however, a set number of criteria on the person specification, and a limited number of ways of posing the questions. Therefore, it is possible to predict the themes and questions likely to be asked. Accordingly, it is possible to start thinking about responses many months in advance of the application form 'going live'. You should consider how to complete 'Homework' questions in this book (marked with the icon and with blank fields for completion) at the end of each relevant chapter, to help you prepare long in advance for the submission of your actual form.

4 Creating a winning application

Marc A Gladman, Manoj Ramachandran, and Mark J Portou

Competition for Foundation Programme posts can be fierce, particularly in certain regions of the country. Therefore, maximizing your score on the 'white space' questions in the online application (see end of Chapter 3) is crucial in two respects: it may ensure that you gain entry to your preferred Foundation school and, further, that you get the particular rotation that you desire.

> ⚠️ **Remember that you are in competition not only with the medical students in your own school and those across the UK, but also with medical students and some qualified doctors from across Europe and beyond! Your application for any particular post therefore requires careful consideration.**

Maximizing your scores

Clearly, achieving the highest possible score is a key factor in determining whether your application to a school's Foundation Programme, and a specific rotation, is successful. Before you attempt to complete your application, it is important that you understand how it will be scored.

For each application, there is a maximum total of 100 points. This is made up of two separate scores; the proportions of each have been changed for the 2009 process:

(1) your academic score (maximum 40 points)

(2) your application form score (maximum 60 points).

1. Academic score

If you are a UK undergraduate, your academic score is calculated automatically by your medical school, and is supplied directly to your local deanery, which will enter it into a national database.

Each year group is divided into four quartiles, based on academic performance, and the score that you receive is determined by which quartile you fall into, as follows:

- first quartile, 40 points

- second quartile, 38 points

- third quartile, 36 points

- fourth quartile, 34 points.

Changes to the 2009 process means that according to this ranking, students in the top 25% of the year (i.e. the first quartile) only have a 6-point advantage over those in the bottom 25% of the year (i.e. the fourth quartile). It is important for those in the fourth quartile to realize that this deficit is not insurmountable if their scores are maximized on the application form. Equally, it is crucial for students in the top quartile not to become complacent and drop marks on the application form, and potentially be 'caught and passed' by those in lower quartiles.

For non-UK graduates or for medical students graduating from a UK medical school before 31 July 2006, the medical school's dean will be asked to provide details of your academic ranking to the Eligibility Office, through which you will have already applied.

2. Application form score

The application form is completed online, is standardized, and carries the majority of the marks. Further, most candidates will be *unable* to alter their academic scores when they come to apply for a Foundation Programme post, as this score reflects performance measured during several years of undergraduate training.

- The application form score is the only variable that you can influence to improve (or worsen!) your application.

- Maximizing your score for each of the 'white space' questions on the form is crucial to achieving a high overall score for an application.

How application form responses are scored

Once your completed form is submitted, it will be marked by a scoring panel, who will allocate marks for each individual answer. It is customary for the panel to consist of a pair of scorers. One is usually a qualified medical doctor and the other a 'lay' representative. It is crucial, therefore, that you avoid unnecessary medical jargon.

Obviously, the details of the marking scheme are confidential. It would be inappropriate, therefore, for any specific details relating to this to be divulged. Furthermore, the marking scheme varies from year to year and thus there is no value in discussing marking schemes from previous years. That said, it is important to appreciate that the scorers will be looking out for certain indicators when marking responses. Some (desirable factors) will increase your score, while others (undesirable factors) will decrease it. The relative proportion of each of these factors will determine your overall score. The obvious aim is to provide the scorers with as many of the desirable and as few of the undesirable factors as possible, to maximize your score for each question.

General approach to completing the form

When you begin to tackle the form, you should consider the five Ps:

- *Prepare* the material – have the questions and person specifications available.

- *Pensive* – think long and hard for the best and most original example.

- *Plan* how to structure each answer.

- *Produce* a draft – this will (dramatically!) exceed the word count.

- *Perfect* – reduce to comply with the word count, and check the grammar and syntax.

The questions are usually available several weeks before the application process opens. You can, therefore, get ahead of the competition by starting well in advance. Although others may appear to be blasé about their application, rest assured that, privately, they will be taking it very seriously. Remember, you are in direct competition with your peers. You should cancel any holidays, lock yourself away for 3 weeks, and concentrate only on your application. Time is short once the process opens. You should aim to perfect your answers so that not a single word is wasted. The early drafts will almost certainly be well over the word limit but in any case needlessly wordy. Each subsequent draft should improve on the last until every single available point is picked up. You should aim to redraft each answer at least five times and perhaps as many as ten or more.

- The form *will* take longer to complete than you initially envisaged – do *not* leave it until the night before the closing date!

- The form *will* need amending and require several drafts.

- You *will* make basic errors – so use a spell-check, and get trusted friends and colleagues to proofread for errors of syntax and grammar.

Approach to individual questions on the form

There are six key considerations when preparing responses. You should do the following:

(1) Read the question and answer everything that is asked
(2) Choose your examples like a 'PRO'
(3) Be precise and concise, correct spellings, and use 'power verbs'
(4) Use a structure, such as the SPAR technique
(5) Sell yourself
(6) Tell the truth.

1. Read the question and answer everything that is asked

Answer *exactly* what the question is asking, and do not be tempted to answer a different question. This sounds obvious, but all too often applicants write the response to a question that they wished they had been asked rather than the one that was actually asked! It is often helpful when planning your response to break the question down into its constituent parts. For example:

Give one example of a non-academic achievement, and explain both its significance to you and its relevance to Foundation training.

This question (Chapter 6) can be broken down into three parts:

- *one* example of a *non-academic* achievement
- its significance *to you*
- its *relevance* to Foundation training.

2. Choose your examples like a 'PRO'

The questions on the form are seeking to determine whether you possess specific skills and qualities required of Foundation Programme doctors, as set out in the person specification (see Appendix). So, if you are asked to provide an example of team working, try to identify one specific example that demonstrates both a team approach and your ability to work in a team. You must avoid the temptation to talk about your general experience when you are asked to give *specific* examples. Examples with clearly defined outcomes tend to work better, particularly those that have a positive outcome.

The examples that you choose for each of the questions should satisfy the PRO criteria:

- *Personal* – delve into your personal experience.

- *Relevant* – it must demonstrate the skill or quality being asked of in the question.

- *Original* – come up with something that won't be used by your peers (competitors!). This is your chance to impress the marker.

⚠️ **Examples to avoid at all costs are those that:**

- **will not be understood by laypeople**

- **many others will use (e.g. giving examples of experience on multidisciplinary or cardiac arrest teams in response to questions about team working)**

- **are too negative or attribute blame to others**

- **are above your level of medical experience (e.g. a medical student/Foundation doctor would not be expected to decide to take a patient to the operating theatre!).**

3. Be precise and concise, correct spellings, and use 'power verbs'

The number of words that you are allowed to use for each of your responses is limited on the form. Many applicants see this as a disadvantage, but it actually encourages the construction of concise sentences. However, ensure that you precisely provide responses to each component of the question. There is no excuse for grammatical errors or spelling mistakes when completing the form. You response may be marked down for such errors. Computer spell-checks are not always accurate or sufficient; get your finished article proofread by someone else.

Passive descriptions will have far less impact than sentences that use active or 'power' verbs. Power verbs such as 'accomplished', 'negotiated', and 'facilitated' will give your sentences a great deal more impact than 'completed', 'arranged', and 'helped' (see also Chapter 12).

4. Use a structure, such as the SPAR technique

A clear structure to your answer is essential. A well-structured answer not only makes identification of key points easier for the markers, guaranteeing that you receive all the marks that you deserve, but also ensures that you address, and thus score, points for *every* section of the question. The acronym SPAR is useful for this purpose:

- *Situation*

- *Problem*

- *Action*

- *Result/reflection/relevance* to Foundation training.

Situation

The situation sets the scene for the rest of the answer, and details your chosen example. You should very briefly but *clearly* describe your example, keeping it relevant to the question. The description should be precise and concise, and should focus only on those details that are pertinent to your answer. Avoid waffling, as this creates a bad first impression and consumes words that will be needed later on.

Problem

Having succinctly described your situation, it is useful to define the specific problem that needed to be addressed. This section together with the situation section should account for approximately one-third of the word allocation.

Action

This section describes what *you* did. Usually, this section accounts for approximately another third of the word allocation. You should concentrate on demonstrating those personal skills, attributes, and characteristics that are required of Foundation Programme doctors, as set out in the person specification. Consider what actions or power verbs describe the clinical or personal skill being evaluated (e.g. team working), rather than simply repeatedly mentioning that skill!

Result/reflection/relevance to Foundation training

Ideally, your example should have a positive and definite outcome that can be accurately described. Try to draw relevant conclusions from the example. More importantly, marks are available for reflections on what you have learned, and how this knowledge is relevant and applicable to Foundation training.

Omission of the last two elements above is the main reason for applicants dropping marks – address them in every question to maximize the marks that you are awarded.

5. Sell yourself

This may sound obvious, but, unless otherwise specified, the question is aimed at evaluating your personal skills, attributes, and characteristics, all of which you will utilize fully as a Foundation Programme doctor. Do not be tempted to appear self-effacing or to undervalue your own contributions for the sake of modesty. Remember, this application form is *your* sales pitch. Only *you* can sell yourself.

 You must sell yourself but be careful not to overstep the line between confidence and arrogance.

6. Tell the truth

Do not be tempted to fabricate examples or embellish them to make them sound more impressive. Likewise, exaggerating your role in any given situation should be avoided. Don't forget that one of the scorers will be a medical doctor, and so will be fully aware what is appropriate for your level of training.

Anyone even suspected of submitting an invalid or falsified response will have their application referred on to the chief assessor, which may then lead on to referral to the central authorities.

Q: What are the most crucial considerations to ensure that I achieve high scores for my responses?

A: You must:
  • provide clear and relevant examples
  • demonstrate clear evidence of reflection/learning
  • appreciate how your experience will be relevant to Foundation training.

Q: What annoys the scorers the most and will result in me achieving poor scores?

A: They get most annoyed by:
  • spelling and grammatical mistakes
  • poor or irrelevant examples
  • too many words given to describing the example
  • a lack of learning from or reflection on the situation
  • failure to explain the relevance to Foundation training.

Golden tips for a successful Foundation application (courtesy of Sukhjinder Nijjer and Jasdeep Gill):

- Set aside plenty of time to prepare and construct your answers.

- Complete the application form in stages.

- Save each section as you go along.

- Always read the question carefully and highlight key words.

- Select your examples carefully – consider which example will display your skills best.

- Avoid repetition and do not use the same example twice.

- Ensure that you answer every part of the question.

- Be concise and keep within the word limit.

- Proofread your answers.

- Check for spelling and grammar mistakes.

- Copy and paste your answers very carefully if you construct your answers offline.

- Print out a hard copy and recheck it.

- Submit your application form as early as possible to allow for any website glitches.

- Breathe a huge sigh of relief and relax!

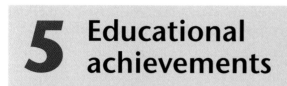

5 Educational achievements

Elena Nikiphorou

In previous years, one question has related to educational achievements, for which a variable number of points (usually four or five) have been available. Usually, the instruction within this question is to *list* these achievements. Consequently, this is the only section in the entire form where lists are permissible, although some applicants may wish to expand their responses.

 Q: List your educational achievements (250 words).

Clarity is crucial when answering this question. In previous years, the guidance notes to the application form have suggested structuring the response to this question in two parts, with marks being available for each.

1. Additional degrees

First, details of any additional degrees to your primary medical qualification should be listed. An intercalated BSc is a common example. The additional qualifications carry different weights, depending on the *level* and *class* obtained. A typical marking scheme, used in previous years, is summarized in Table 5.1.

Table 5.1. A typical marking scheme for additional qualifications

Points	Educational achievement	
0	None mentioned (blank box), or non-educational achievement given	
1	BSc or BA Class unspecified or third class or equivalent	
2	BSc or BA Class 2:2	
3	BSc or BA Class 2:1	Masters degree
4	BSc or BA Class 1st	PhD or doctorate

It is crucial that you provide the class achieved in your degree, as this will affect the score that you receive. The maximum number of points that you can score for this part of the question is 4.

2. Additional academic achievements

The second part of the answer focuses on any additional academic achievements, such as national prizes, publications, and presentations. The maximum score available is usually only 1, so don't panic if you do not have any! If you are fortunate enough to have secured such achievements, they should be listed as detailed below.

Prizes

Previously, only *national* prizes have received marks in this section, although it is worth listing any awarded at regional or local level, in case discretionary marks are available. If you have any, you should state the name or title of the prize, the organization awarding it, and what it was. Try to list the date last, as this is usually the least important detail (see also Chapter 13). Example responses might be:

National Mathematics Competition. Awarded to the top-ranking student in mathematics in an open competition across the UK. Awarded by the London Mathematical Society (2005).

National Medical Student Prize for the Best Abstract of the Year. Subject: Abstract on the most important development in medicine over the last decade. Awarded by Imperial College (2004).

It is good to give numbers in this section if possible. For example, winning a prize when 200 students entered a competition is more impressive than if there were only 5 competitors.

Publications

Any publications in national or international peer-reviewed journals, where you are a named contributor, should be included. These should be listed using the Vancouver style format (see example below). Essential information when citing a journal article include:

- list of authors (name, initials)
- title of article
- name of journal (abbreviated form and in italics)

- year/month of publication
- volume/issue number (in bold)
- page numbers.

For example:

Alan K, Franks MP, Stevens A. Medical ethics, communication and learning. *Med Educ* 1998; **325**: 24–8.

Jones A, Smith LJ. The latest developments in medical sciences. *BMJ* 2000; **234**: 145–8.

Q: What if my paper has not been published yet but is due out soon?

A: You need to have evidence that the paper has been accepted for publication. The recognized way of doing this is to quote a PMID number (this can be found listed below your paper-to-be on common databases such as PubMed).

Do not list papers that you are currently writing or that are under review by a journal. These are not publications as yet and, if the scorers decide to check, there will be no record of your paper even existing. This is almost as if you have lied – so be careful!

Presentations

Any oral or poster presentations at national or international meetings or conferences should be mentioned here. You should preferably be the first or second named author. The details listed for such presentations will be similar to those listed for a publication, but with the journal name being substituted by the name of the conference or meeting at which the presentation was given. For example:

Brown K, Andrews P. Calcium metabolism and the kidney. Royal Society of Medicine, London, June 2006.

Vasudevan SP, Swash M, Lunniss PJ, Scott SM. Is the rectal contractile response to distension altered in patients with rectal hyposensitivity? International Neurogastroenterology and Motility Meeting, Boston, USA, September 2006.

Q: If I presented at a departmental meeting in my local hospital as a medical student, does this count as a presentation?

A: If you have no other presentations, or if it was a particularly interesting talk that may catch the eye of the scorer, then it is worth listing a local or regional presentation. Do note, however, that it is up to the scorer whether to give you marks for such an entry.

- Remember that you may be asked to produce proof of all your educational achievements, so do not be tempted to lie!

- Even if you do not have any additional degrees or academic achievements, you will miss out on relativity few marks – so don't get disheartened!

- Organize your answer using headings, as this helps to show that you have a methodical approach to your thinking and work.

- To take your answer a step further, try to personally reflect on what you learnt. A relatively basic achievement can score highly if you demonstrate its significance and your personal development resulting from it.

Example answers

To finish off this chapter, let's look at a poor example and a good example when answering this question (examples courtesy of Jas Gill).

Poor answer

Medicine degree – passed years 1–4, no re-sits.

Prize: the 'Here You Go' bursary for my elective project in Year 4.

Publication in the Journal of Infection on handwashing & MRSA among healthcare professionals in May 2006.

Publication in the student British Medical Journal on coping under pressure in June 2007.

Research into 'Awareness of handwashing & MRSA among healthcare professionals' on a cohort of 300.

Audit on 'Use of proton-pump inhibitors in patients on NSAIDS'.

Presented 'Case report – Liver disease' at Hospital of London Grand Round.

Good answer

Degrees
MBChB – ranked in second quartile.
Distinctions in 2 out of 5 modules in Year 4.

Prizes
Awarded the 'Here You Go' bursary from University of London for my elective project in Year 4 by competitive application and interview.

Publications
Student A. Hand-washing among healthcare professionals. Journal of Infection 2006; **123**: 123–124.
Student A. Coping under pressure. Student BMJ 2007; **123**: 12–13.

Research
Cross-sectional study on a cohort of 300 healthcare professionals into their awareness of hand-washing & MRSA. I successfully secured funding from London Hospital Trust and ethical approval. The findings were presented regionally and published in the Journal of Infection.

Audit

Audit on 'Use of proton-pump inhibitors in patients on NSAIDS' at London General Practice, which I independently organized, conducted, and presented.

Presentations

Presented 'Awareness of hand-washing and MRSA among healthcare professionals' at Hospital of London, 2007 – awarded best student presentation.

Presented 'Use of proton–pump inhibitors in patients on NSAIDS' to doctors and nurses at London General Practice, 2006.

Presented 'Case report – Liver disease' at Hospital of London Grand Round, 2006.

Through my numerous achievements, I have learnt to manage and prioritize my time effectively to balance my academic and personal success. I take the initiative and am reliable in my work. I hope to develop my skills further during my Foundation training.

This second answer displays the level of involvement and achievement more clearly. It is more logical and easier to read at a glance. There is also a short reflection at the end which demonstrates self-appraisal skills.

List your educational achievements.

6 Non-academic achievements

Mark J Portou, Manoj Ramachandran, and Marc A Gladman

Medical school is an opportunity for you to broaden your horizons, have new experiences, and excel in aspects of life other than academia, in addition to studying to become a doctor. Modern selection processes for medical school have been designed to recruit more rounded individuals.

Referring to the person specification (see Appendix), most of the characteristics outlined as essential qualities of Foundation Programme doctors are by no means specific to medicine. For example, among the personal skills listed are:

- the ability to prioritize tasks and information appropriately
- an understanding of the importance of working effectively with others
- the ability to communicate effectively with colleagues
- the ability to deal effectively with pressure and/or challenge.

Application form questions on non-academic achievements are an opportunity for you to show that you possess these skills and that you can translate them to the start of your medical career (i.e. Foundation training). These questions have consistently appeared on previous application forms.

Q: *Give an example of a non-academic achievement, and explain both its significance to you and its relevance to Foundation training. (150 words)*

Q: *How should I break this question down when planning my response?*

A: There are three key components to the task:
- identify a *non-academic* example
- explain its significance to *you*
- explain its significance to *Foundation training*.

In the remainder of this chapter we will work through each of these components.

This question clearly specifies only one example, and so you *will* be marked down for giving more than one. The one example used must be non-academic; suitable examples are discussed below.

As long as your chosen achievement is non-academic, the detail of the example is more or less irrelevant. What is crucial to this question is demonstration of why this achievement is *significant*, and in particular why it is significant to *you*, and how it is significant to *Foundation training* (of help here may be the SPAR technique described in Chapter 4).

1. Identify a suitable example of a non-academic achievement

There are two considerations here. First, the example described must be non-academic. Second, it should be an achievement.

Make sure that your example demonstrates an actual *achievement*. Writing about being awarded a badge for swimming 25 m is unlikely to impress the scorers marking your application! Similarly, choosing examples that apply to all applicants, such as getting into medical school, hardly sets you aside from the crowd.

Non-academic examples

You can choose any non-academic achievement. It does not have to be spectacular. Most people will not have won an Olympic gold medal, had a hit album, or won a Nobel Peace Prize. As long as you explain how and why the example chosen is an achievement, you will score the points.

Suitable examples for non-academic achievements include:

- sporting achievements

- musical achievements

- committee work

- organizing events

- voluntary work

- election to positions of responsibility

- situations in which you have overcome adversity.

Ensure that something is achieved

Achievement can be defined as the act of accomplishing or finishing successfully, especially by means of exertion, skill, practice, or perseverance.

In order for your example to be suitable, it should demonstrate a clear end-point. Without evidence of goal or task completion, or the accomplishment of a positive outcome, it cannot really be considered an achievement.

2. Explain its significance to you

Once you have identified a suitable example of an achievement (perhaps from the list of examples above), its significance to you can be considered, based around any of the following:

- What was *significant* about this achievement?
- What was the *personal* significance of the achievement?
- How did this role/situation *challenge* you?
- How was the *outcome successful*?
- What did you *learn*?

Demonstrating that you learned something – either as a result of the outcome or in the process of reaching that outcome – is crucial in this question and many others on the application form. Evidence of learning can be presented in two ways:

- specific skills
- generic skills.

Specific skills

Specific skills will relate to the outcome itself (i.e. the achievement) and will be derived from the end-point. An example would be describing the upper-body strength and climbing skills developed while mountaineering. Clearly, relating these particular skills to the Foundation Programme will take a lot of imagination! Therefore, as a general rule, it is better to give examples involving specific skills that can easily and obviously be demonstrated during daily practice, as these are likely to score higher.

Generic skills

Generic skills are those developed and practised in the process of completing the achievement. They are transferable skills that, although extremely important in task-specific achievements, will also apply in many daily situations. Using the above extreme example of mountain climbing, reference to the planning and organization, teamwork, and trust from colleagues necessary to complete the task will be far more impressive and will score more highly.

Key generic skills include:

- leadership

- team working

- responsibility/trust

- communication

- time management

- competence

- organization

- negotiation

- public speaking/presentation

- teaching

- learning

- meeting deadlines.

There will be many others of course, but your answer should include only those relevant to your achievement, to make your answer more individual, even unique.

3. Explain its significance to Foundation training

As mentioned above, reference to generic, transferable skills will make the process of relating your achievement and what you learned from it much easier. Just look at the list on page 65 again. Each one of those generic skills applies to the daily practice of Foundation Programme doctors. Therefore, relating these to their use in Foundation training should be simple.

A structured answer is essential. Use the SPAR technique when planning your answer (see Chapter 4). A worked example showing how this can be effective is given below.

Summary of general principles

- Structure your answer using the SPAR technique.

- The example must have a clear end-point.

- What did you do/what was your role?

- What did you learn?

- Generic skills are better than specific.

- Mention must be made of the achievement's relevance to Foundation training.

Example answers

Poor answer

For my elective, I undertook a hospital placement in Tanzania. While travelling through the country, I met lots of interesting people and enjoyed many new experiences. A group of people I met offered me the chance to join their expedition to climb Mount Kilimanjaro, and we set off a week later. This was a big achievement for me as I had never done anything like this before, and it was very physically demanding. The expedition tested my fitness to the extreme and required me to use all my upper-body strength and stamina. I also had to contend with very little sleep and a lot of blisters, as well as the very cold weather. This experience gave me an enormous sense of achievement.

This answer will score poorly. While the example may be impressive, the answer fails to explain the personal significance of this achievement, and offers no reflection or evidence of learning. The relevance to the Foundation Programme has also been completely overlooked.

It is obvious from this extreme example that an impressive achievement is no guarantee of a good score, and more modest examples will score much better if they show evidence of reflection, learning, and relevance to the Foundation Programme, rather than simply telling a story.

Better answer

> *I have always had an interest in coaching football. After 1-year of training and practice, I was awarded the level 3 licence in coaching by the Football Association. It included studying (and being examined on) subjects such as child protection, sports psychology, management of sports injuries, and basic life support. I had to plan and deliver these coaching sessions for large groups while being assessed. It required me to work closely with, and observe, senior coaches, and to personally arrange these placements. I researched subjects I was unfamiliar with, using a variety of sources. The course required effective time management skills in order to dedicate sufficient time to its study, while balancing the demands of an undergraduate medical course. On gaining this licence, I felt an enormous sense of pride and achievement.*

Although this is a better example, there is still room for improvement. There is little structure and most of the answer refers to the process of gaining the achievement. The evidence of learning is weak and, while some of the key skills are mentioned, they are not tied in to the relevance to Foundation training.

Good answer

[Situation]
Determined to obtain recognition for my interest in coaching football, after a gruelling year of training and practice, I was awarded the Football Association level 3 coaching licence.

[Problem]
The course required effective time management skills while balancing the demands of an undergraduate medical course. I studied subjects such as child protection, sports psychology, management of sports injuries, and basic life support, arranging each placement individually.

[Action]
This achievement utilized and honed my skills of negotiation, through effective communication, and I developed leadership and teamwork skills in order to command the attention of groups of varying age and ability. I researched unfamiliar subjects in order to achieve the required level of competence.

[Result]
Achieving this award has direct relevance for the Foundation Programme, as teaching skills are fundamental to good medical practice. The ability to learn independently, and to find valid sources of information and reference, is essential to the Foundation years and beyond.

This answer, clearly structured using the SPAR technique (as flagged, but not of course included in the actual submission), shows evidence of learning from the process, and the relevance to the Foundation programme is made explicit.

Give an example of a non-academic achievement, and explain both its significance to you and its relevance to Foundation training. (150 words)

Example:

Significance:

Relevance:

7 Coping under pressure

Sukhjinder Nijjer and Jasdeep Gill

Pressure exists in our everyday lives and you will have already experienced significant pressure during your time at medical school. Understanding and coping with pressure is an essential part of all doctors' lives. Being able to cope with pressure is a critical skill that will serve you and your future patients. The Royal Colleges, the PMETB (Postgraduate Medical Education and Training Board), and the GMC all recognize 'coping with pressure' as an essential criterion during recruitment of doctors at all stages of their careers. Therefore, being able to demonstrate on the application form that you can cope with pressure is critical.

As a Foundation doctor, you will face a wide range of pressures, from having to deal with too many patients at once to developing your medical career while maintaining your social life. The latter has, until recently, been somewhat neglected as a priority. However, the Department of Health now recognizes the need for increased emphasis on establishing a healthy work–life balance.

Answering questions on 'coping with pressure' can be difficult at this early stage in your career. This chapter will discuss how to cope with pressure and how to tackle these questions using real-life personal examples. You may have developed a number of coping mechanisms subconsciously. Some of these will be good and others bad. We will discuss ideal coping mechanisms that you can use, not only on a daily basis, but also to stimulate ideas for your answers on the application form.

The inverted J-shaped curve

Stress and pressure have a number of benefits, and successful people are able to use them to their advantage. Under mild stress, you can become more organized, more productive, work more efficiently, concentrate more, and neglect unimportant tasks. You will have already dealt with numerous stressful episodes and experienced the benefits of stress to reach this point in your career. As a Foundation doctor, you will have many stressors that drive you to work to your best ability. However, too much stress can have an adverse effect, and can even cause psychological and physical harm. You may become less productive, grouchy, and irritable, and perhaps behave irrationally and out of character. These are clearly undesirable traits for a doctor, who should remain calm and in control during times of stress and pressure. While you may not feel it, others will be looking to you for direction and support during difficult times.

This property of stress has been described in terms of an inverted J-shaped curve (Figure 7.1). Your aim is to achieve maximum productivity at a mild or intermediate level of stress, without being crippled by high levels of stress. The way that you cope

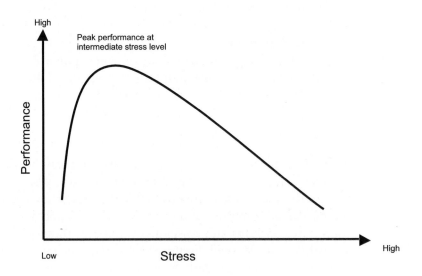

Figure 7.1. The inverted J-shaped curve of stress versus performance.

with stress will determine the inflection point on the curve. By recognizing stress and responding appropriately, you can move yourself to a preferable part of the curve.

Biologically, the body responds to stress with both sympathetic activation (the 'flight or fight' response) and cortisol release. While helpful in the short term, prolonged levels of high cortisol suppress the immune system and decrease resistance to ill health and disease.

Physical and psychological effects of stress

- **Decreased stamina**

- **Sleep problems (e.g. increased need for sleep or insomnia)**

- **Weight loss or gain; decreased or increased appetite**

- **Proneness to accidents**

- **Increased susceptibility to illness**

- **Psychosomatic complaints (e.g. headaches, migraines, ulcers, or backaches)**

- **Substance misuse – excessive drinking or drug use**

- **Cardiopulmonary problems (e.g. increased blood pressure or heart disease)**

- **Depression, mood changes, or crying easily**

- **Isolation – lack of desire to socialize or simply isolating yourself from others, either physically or emotionally**

- **Marital/family conflicts**

- **Cynicism**

- **Aggression**

- **Self-esteem problems – sense of despair, emptiness, or worthlessness**

Effects of stress on work and health

The Health and Safety Executive has identified that stress and pressure at work account for over one-third of all new episodes of ill health. Each case of work-related stress-, depression-, or anxiety-related ill health leads to an average of 30.2 lost working days. A total of 13.8 million working days were lost to work-related stress, depression, and anxiety in 2006–7.

Doctors are notoriously bad at recognizing their own ill health and often neglect themselves in order 'to get the job done'. Recent changes in medical training, the European Working Time Directive, and a noticeable change in the structure of the medical team appear to have reduced the medical fraternity's levels of stress and pressure. However, these changes in themselves have introduced new pressures, and the need for adaptive coping mechanisms remains.

Identifying stressors

Picture yourself as a Foundation doctor. Look critically at the day-to-day tasks performed and the approaches used to solve problems. You will find some tasks appear very stressful for the uninitiated and yet are easy for more senior doctors. Experience makes a big difference to how you view a task and how you cope with the pressure that the task generates. However, there are many other factors that interact to modify the stress generated. If you can identify the key factors, you can reduce the stress and therefore be more productive. Try to think of a list of 'stressors' that would plague your life as a junior doctor, as this will give you an insight into answering a question on coping with pressure. These could be categorized into professional and personal factors, as on page 75.

A sample list of 'stressors' experienced by junior doctors

Professional factors

- Unwell patients

- Not enough experience or skills

- Lack of time to perform tasks

- Lack of knowledge to perform tasks

- Lack of teamwork

- Lack of control over your environment and the demands placed upon you

- Poor relationship with team members or consultant

- Unrealistic expectations from team or seniors

- Communication difficulties with patients or staff

- Unhelpful management or administration

- Rota difficulties

- Seeking perfection (overly high self-expectation)

- Feelings of you against 'the system'

- NHS and hospital politics

Personal factors

- Insufficient leisure time

- Family and social demands on time

- Living arrangements

- Financial worries

- Child-care issues

- Commuting to work

Take the opportunity to look at a stressful time in your life. Are there similarities between this time and what you might expect your experience as a Foundation doctor will be? Try to divide the stressful time into its key components, and assign each factor a score of importance (e.g. out of 10). By doing this, you are already beginning to break down the problem and prioritize the tasks. This will help you see the situation in context and reduce the associated stress, and will help you cope.

It is also important to recognize that medical students and doctors are high achievers. You are used to success and may well have a very 'driven' personality. This increases your likelihood of experiencing stress and suffering burnout. Seeking perfection is admirable but often not possible within our complex healthcare system. Learning that the 'best possible care' does not mean 'perfection' will help reduce your stress levels.

Coping strategies

There are many unhealthy and maladaptive strategies to cope with pressure. You will recognize some or all of these in yourself or among your friends and colleagues.

Unhealthy ways of coping under pressure

- **Chain smoking**

- **Self-medicating with alcohol or drugs**

- **Procrastinating**

- **Withdrawing from friends, family, and activities**

- **Eating too much or too little**

- **Sleeping too much or too little**

- **Avoiding the pressure by pretending it's not there**

- **Self-pity and complaining**

Before we explore the question of how to cope with pressure, the following general tips are for your personal use when trying to cope under pressure at work.

How to cope under pressure

- Recognize fatigue

- Find time for regular relaxation and sleep

- Take breaks

- Monitor your state of mind; become aware of stress indicators

- Manage your time by being more organized and by prioritizing.

- Be flexible and keen to change if things are not working

- Ensure that you are given space and time for personal development and continuous education

- Develop teams and a network of support

- Have a healthy diet

- Find time for activities or hobbies that you really enjoy

- Celebrate success and accomplishment

- Book annual leave in advance and organize a holiday – and look forward to it!

Some but not all of these will help you. We are all unique and people cope in different ways. Spend time reflecting on your personality and your own coping strategies. What has helped you succeed? What has hindered you? Taking a reflective approach is important in coping with stress, as it allows you to move along the adult learning cycle. If a strategy worked, why did it help and how could it be improved?

Conceptualize new ways of coping and introduce them to your repertoire. Reflect again on whether they worked and then modify accordingly. In this way, you can treat dealing with stress as you would any other task, and you can get better at dealing with it.

Stressors in the workplace can quickly pile on top of each other. Learn the skills that you need to cope with them as they arise.

How to cope with 'stressors'

- Recognize the stress and identify why it is a stressor

- Make specific time to prioritize tasks

- Tackle the most important tasks immediately

- Recognize your limits

- Seek the help of a more senior doctor early

- Open clear communication channels with team members and nursing staff

- Make an appointment with your consultant to discuss your concerns

- Discuss issues with your educational supervisor or pastoral advisor

Prioritization is an essential skill for all doctors, and will help you cope with pressure. It is often easier to prioritize your personal tasks. Knowing how to prioritize your tasks as a Foundation doctor will require experience. You may need guidance and support from a more senior doctor, particularly when dealing with sick patients, and some apparently unimportant tasks may take precedence owing to administrative processes in your hospital. Setting aside time specifically to prioritize your tasks should form an integral part of your day.

Good time management goes hand in hand with prioritization. Conserve as much time as possible; use a schedule but do not follow it slavishly. Be in control of your time; learn to say 'no' to unimportant tasks and delegate those better performed by others. Make time by focusing on priorities, reorganizing them as things change. Always do what is urgent first.

Keep a log-book of the patients whom you have seen, times of stress, and how you coped. Identify your strengths and areas for improvement. Do not be too hard on yourself; you are still learning and even very experienced doctors are still learning to cope with pressure.

Dealing with emotional stresses

Healthcare is an emotive arena and there will have been times when a patient's situation has been emotionally challenging. Doctors must recognize and acknowledge the effect of emotional stress on their lives. Some mask their stress and front it out by putting on a brave face. For many, this can be counterproductive. Discuss your feelings with a colleague or another confidant(e). Discussing difficulties with non-medical friends may also help, provided that patient confidentiality is maintained. Many hospitals have patient advisory liaison services (PALS), which are designed to help patients and relatives cope with issues arising during illness. Many of these services are also willing to help stressed members of staff. Other hospitals have a chaplaincy service or a staff counsellor. Seeking professional help can be a mature way of dealing with stresses before they affect your health or performance.

Dealing with personal stresses

Trying to find the perfect balance between work and personal life is stressful in itself. Finding time for yourself and your partner, family, and friends while working in a busy post can be difficult. Attempting to do it all can lead to anxiety, fatigue, and burnout. It is not possible for everyone to do everything, and even those who appear to have everything will have stress that is unknown to you. Prioritization and identifying what is important to you are essential. Discuss your stresses with your family and friends.

They may be able to help with even apparently insurmountable tasks and help you see things in context.

As you grow older, your priorities will change. Actively developing your own philosophy and world view will give you a perspective on day-to-day and longer-term stresses. Identify for yourself the highest priority in your life and what you are prepared to do to achieve it. Understanding yourself is key to coping with pressure.

Example questions and answers

Q1: Give an example of a situation when you felt under pressure. How did you manage this, and what did you learn that will be relevant to your Foundation training? (150 words)

There are three distinct parts to this question, and you must address each part. Ensure that you keep referring back to the question as you write your answer, to make sure that you answer it all.

Start off by thinking about potential examples that may be suitable. The example could be from a clinical or non-clinical setting. To help you choose the most suitable example, select the one with a clear and definable outcome, and which allowed you to demonstrate your skills and reflect on what you had learnt. Remember, you will be marked on how you coped under pressure rather than on the situation itself, so overly dramatic examples will not help you to gain marks. Avoid examples that could show yourself or colleagues in a negative light, and avoid criticizing the system or colleagues. Aim to select an example that had a satisfactory outcome. Suitable examples may include dealing with a difficult patient or relative, juggling several deadlines, personal difficulties or setbacks, handling criticism, or feeling out of your depth during a particular task. Whichever example you use, make sure that you show insight into what the problem was, and use it to demonstrate your suitability for Foundation training.

Reflect on and evaluate what you have learnt, because it will add a personal element to your answer. Demonstrate that you can think laterally about a particular situation. In addition, self-appraisal skills are becoming more widely recognized, and specific sections within the Foundation Programme learning portfolio directly focus on appraisal of your own performance.

Example answer

Throughout medical school, I have continued employment as a sales assistant in a local retail shop while successfully balancing my personal and academic life. During end-of-year examinations, I was under enormous pressure to juggle everything. I have learnt to develop my prioritization and time-management skills using comprehensive lists. These skills will be essential throughout Foundation training to ensure that patient needs are prioritized and daily jobs are completed.

If unable to work a shift on the rota, I ensure that I make suitable arrangements for a colleague to cover. This has instilled within me the importance of responsibility and accountability, which are skills that I need for Foundation training.

I often deal with customer complaints and have learnt the importance of customer satisfaction. These skills will be useful to me during my Foundation training when communicating with patients.

This response answers only parts of the question. The example used is very broad, and so the answer is superficial. The candidate uses the sweeping statement 'pressure to juggle everything' but does not unravel or identify what the pressures were. This demonstrates that the candidate lacks the insight to identify the issues. If someone cannot identify the stressors, then they cannot begin to deal with them. It is important for you to identify the pressure(s) clearly and concisely.

This answer does not describe how the candidate managed the pressure. Therefore, a third of the marks are automatically unobtainable. However, the candidate has reflected well on what was learnt from the experience and its relevance to Foundation training.

Q: *What skills should I be demonstrating on a form when answering a question on coping under pressure?*

A: Try to show some or all of the skills listed below, but have quantifiable, definable outcomes to your answers, as opposed to broad statements.
- Prioritization
- Planning
- Organization
- Communication
- Teamwork
- Problem solving
- Delegation
- Responsibility
- Time management
- Negotiation
- Awareness of limitations
- Insight and ability to ask for help
- Judgement
- Accountability

Q2: *Describe one example of how you resolved a difficult problem. What skills did you use, and what solution was reached? Explain its relevance to your Foundation training. (150 words)*

This question does not immediately present itself as a 'coping under pressure' question. When answering the Foundation application questions, you must ask yourself exactly what the question is asking, what skills they expect you to demonstrate, and how these will be relevant to your Foundation training.

The example that you use may be selected from any setting, but you must describe it concisely. Make sure that you clearly display your skills. While it is important to include the outcome or solution, the way in which you reached that end-point is more important, and is what you will be marked on.

Example answer

As Year Representative, I faced pressure to address students' academic and welfare issues and meet report deadlines. Students informed me of their dissatisfaction with the lack of mock examination questions available and demanded that I resolve this.

I acknowledged the problem, reassured the year group, and discussed it with the Year Coordinator. I negotiated access to confidential written student feedback to help produce a report of the students' views, which I presented to staff. I kept the year group updated on progress. The outcome was positive and more questions were made available before our examinations.

This experience enhanced my ability to deal maturely with pressures, using patience and diplomacy, which are skills I will require during Foundation training. I developed skills to prioritize tasks and produce reports to strict deadlines. I discussed problems tactfully in committee meetings while maintaining confidentiality. By keeping the year group informed, I helped to reduce their anxiety, which was essential.

This example answers all three components of the question. In particular, the structure of the answer into three distinct paragraphs helps to highlight this to the marker. The first paragraph succinctly sets the scene and identifies the pressure. The second paragraph describes how the candidate successfully managed the pressure and states the outcome. The candidate demonstrates numerous skills, such as empathy, prioritization, communication skills, interpersonal skills, time management, and professionalism. Further depth is added to the answer in the final paragraph, because it clearly demonstrates the candidate's insight into the skills learnt and the relevance to Foundation training.

This answer is well balanced overall. It correctly dedicates fewer words to describing the situation, because the candidate recognizes that the marker is relatively less interested in what the exact situation was. More focus is given to how the situation was managed and what was learnt from the experience.

Conclusions

Coping under pressure is a life skill that you will call upon throughout your medical career. Always take a moment to reflect and identify the pressures in your life; only then will you be able to begin addressing them. Analyse and modify your coping strategies, and choose the methods that best suit your personality. As a junior doctor, there will be many times when you feel out of your depth, and it is vital that you seek senior input early. Asking for help is a trait of a mature and responsible doctor. Establish a sound support network and aim to achieve a healthy work–life balance in order to help you cope with work pressures.

Q1: Give an example of a situation when you felt under pressure. How did you manage this, and what did you learn that will be relevant to your Foundation training?

Q2: Describe one example of how you resolved a difficult problem. What skills did you use, and what solution was reached? Explain its relevance to your Foundation training?

Q3: What coping strategies do you use when under pressure?

Q4: What skills do you use, and why, when faced with a problem or challenge? List the three skills you consider most important, and say why.

Q5: Describe a situation when you demonstrated your ability to cope under pressure. What did you do well, and what could you have done differently?

8 Prioritization

Shondipon K Laha, Marc A Gladman, and Manoj Ramachandran

'Suppose you were taking a course in parachuting and there were 100 things to do successfully. You correctly identified 99 of these 100 items on the written test. But on your first jump, you couldn't remember how to pull the ripcord – the item you missed. You'd probably earn a posthumous A for the course from most teachers, but it wouldn't bring you back from the dead. If you want to jump safely, worry less about your test score and worry about what's important and what's not. Then learn and do the important things.'

Wess Roberts

Prioritization (and related concepts such as organization and planning) is an important aspect of your day-to-day work. From the first day of your job, you will accumulate a tangled nightmare of tasks. Some people will naturally be able to manage their time efficiently, but most have to learn how to organize themselves.

For a junior doctor, the tasks to be prioritized will generally fall into three categories:

- the clinical needs of the job
- personal needs (linked to family and social life)
- longer-term activities.

At work, you must concentrate on the first of these categories as a priority, but you must always bear the other two in mind.

Clinical needs of the job

At the extreme end, you need to be able to prioritize patients according to their clinical need. Accident and emergency departments have a system in place known as 'triage' (from the French *trier*, meaning 'to sort, sift, or select'). This was initally developed during the Napoleonic wars, when patients would be divided into three groups:

- needs rapid attention to live
- needs attention but will live anyway
- is likely to die with or without attention.

Admittedly, this system has been fine-tuned a little since then (e.g. the Revised Trauma Score) and hopefully your hospital is not quite as busy as the Battle of Waterloo!

Prioritization can also be seen in theatres. For example, the National Confidential Enquiry into Perioperative Deaths (NCEPOD) classifies surgical cases as:

- immediate (life or limb saving)
- urgent (conditions that are life or limb threatening)
- expedited (stable patients with conditions that are not immediately life or limb threatening)
- elective (planned admissions).

Deciding what your tasks are and organizing them

Every day you will be given a continuously updating list of jobs. It is important to keep track of these jobs on paper, and then prioritize them appropriately. Here are three of the most common ways of dealing with this, which you can use when preparing your answers for this genre of question.

1. Pareto's principle

In 1906, Vilfredo Pareto, an economist, noticed that Italian wealth was disproportionately distributed: 20% of the popultation owned 80% of the wealth. Other researchers noted that this '80/20 rule' could be used in a variety of different fields. With reference to your daily work, 20% of what you do produces 80% of your results.

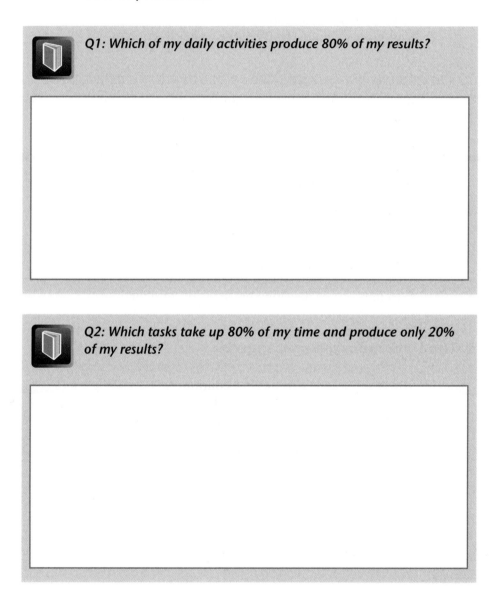

Q1: Which of my daily activities produce 80% of my results?

Q2: Which tasks take up 80% of my time and produce only 20% of my results?

2. The principles of direction, necessity, and efficiency

Another method to define your tasks uses three general principles.

(i) The principle of direction – 'What do I have to achieve?'

Answering this question should allow you:

- to know what your goals and key tasks are
- to identify relevant activities
- to place all your efforts in the right direction.

(ii) The principle of necessity – 'How necessary is this activity?'

Answering this question should allow you:

- to analyse each of the tasks
- to remove unimportant activities
- to concentrate on the important goals.

(iii) The principle of efficiency – 'Am I doing this in the most efficient way?'

Answering this question should allow you:

- to examine the way that you work
- to improve or develop new ways of working.

3. The time management matrix

The use of a time management matrix, such as the one in Figure 8.1, will make clear to you which jobs you need to address first. However, you also need to keep some time free for the second and third boxes.

1. Urgent and important	2. Not urgent but important
• Medical emergencies • Preparing patients for theatre • Some investigations • Preparing presentations for the next day	• Reviewing daily blood tests • Some investigations • Revising for examinations • Filling in application forms • Meals • Extracurricular activities • Holidays
3. Urgent but not important	4. Not urgent and not important
• Some telephone calls and bleeps • Most interruptions • Some meetings	• Watching television • Gossiping

Figure 8.1. The time management matrix, with some example entries for a junior doctor.

All three methods outlined above can work only if you systematically make a job list. It is important to recognize that you may never finish all the tasks that you have set yourself. Taking breaks and time for meals are very important, and may help you to avoid making simple mistakes. It is also important to know when to call for help, especially when patient safety is at stake.

Example questions and answers

 Q1: Describe an example of how your organizational and planning skills have contributed to a significant personal achievement in the last 5 years. What did you learn from this that is relevant to Foundation training?

This is an example of reflective practice: looking for an acomplishment over your time at medical school. In your answer you must be able to demonstrate analysis, reflection, learning, and relevance. This could be done as follows.

- Define your *significant* achievement (e.g. completing dissertations, research projects, or examinations successfully). This question also allows you to look at non-medical achievements (e.g. sporting activities, helping charities, organizing social events, sitting on a representative body).
- Think of the factors that affected how you completed that achievement (e.g. time pressure, other work commitments, social or familial responsibilities). Include the component parts.
- You can use the systems mentioned above to describe how you rationalized those factors and achieved that goal.
- Explain how you would apply what you learnt to Foundation training, either to training as a whole or to specific situations (e.g. to your future workload, your own education, performing audit, taking on research, or maintaining a healthy work–life balance).

Poor answer

In my 4th year, I was posted to the surgical ward at my teaching hospital. During the 3 months that I was there, I noticed that none of the patients seemed to have any idea of why they were still in hospital, and when they could expect to leave. I conducted an audit of all the patients who came in over 4 weeks, by myself, and presented it to the consultants. This required me to organize a meeting for consultants, design the audit form, and get authorization to conduct the study from my supervisor. The result was that the consultant staff realized that they had to be much clearer in communicating their treatment intentions to their patients. This ability to organize will be very useful for the Foundation years, as I can not only organize the daily tests needed for my patients, but also participate in audits to improve the quality of their care.

This answer shows a complete lack of insight into what the question is asking for. Not only is this *not* a significant achievement, but it also portrays an individual working in the system, laying blame (in an unprofessional manner) on senior colleagues, and single-handedly trying to sort out the problems perceived to exist!

Good answer

I initiated, and individually managed, an 'aerobics marathon' in central London, raising in excess of £3000 towards the Save Every Single Dog Fund and increasing awareness about homeless dogs.

I multi-tasked and led on individual tasks such as police clearance for street collections, equipment hire, insurance, T-shirt printing, local advertising, and radio broadcasting. I successfully persuaded 30 team members to offer their services over a 12-hour period to keep the aerobics machines running, and to collect money from the general public. I have since been nominated for my college's student union 'social colours' award for coordinating the event.

I have improved my ability to communicate clearly and to achieve complex tasks outside a medical environment. Learning to prioritize my tasks while ensuring that they are all completed efficiently and fluently, within an allocated time, will help me greatly in my Foundation training post.

In this answer, there is certainly a significant and quantifiable personal achievement, made possible using multiple individual skills that the applicant has clearly demonstrated. The answer is made more comprehensive by bringing in related skills such as leadership and team-working capabilities. Finally, these past achievements are tied in to the future Foundation training post. There are, however, other aspects to planning, organization, and prioritization that could have been included.

ORGANISE (courtesy of Marc A Gladman)

This acronym will help you to remember all the important aspects of an answer to any question involving prioritization, organization, and/or planning.

Other plans (contingencies)

Risk management

Goal setting

Ability to prioritize

Numerous tasks (multi-tasking)

Improves methodology

Sticks to time

Evaluates success/failure

Q2: Describe one example from your undergraduate medical training of your ability to prioritize tasks and information from any clinical or education area. What was the outcome, what have you learned, and how will you apply this to Foundation training?

This is similar to the previous question, but does not include the scope to look at non-medical areas.

- Define your example (an achievement such as passing examinations with honours, organizing a teaching session, or completing an audit or research project).
- Think of the tasks and information needed to achieve this.
- Use the systems above to demonstrate how you prioritized to achieve the outcome.
- Discuss the outcome. It is less important whether the outcome was successful or not; however, you need to demonstrate how it developed your prioritization skills.
- Again, use this information to demonstrate how you would apply this to Foundation training.

Q1: Describe a situation in which you have had a number of things to be done at the same time. How did you approach that situation, and what was the result? How will you apply this to Foundation training?

Q2: Describe an example of how your organizational and planning skills have contributed to a significant personal achievement in the last 5 years. What did you learn from this that is relevant to Foundation training?

Q3: Describe one example from your undergraduate medical training of your ability to prioritize tasks and information from any clinical or education area. What was the outcome, what have you learned, and how will you apply this to Foundation training?

9 Team working and leadership

Shalini Kawar and
Manoj Ramachandran

Application forms may assess both team-working and leadership skills, and therefore knowledge of the skills involved, and how to differentiate between them, will identify the more successful candidates.

Team working

A team can be defined as a small number of people with complementary skills who are committed to a common purpose, performance goals, and approach, for which they are mutually accountable. The GMC's document *Duties of a Doctor* (General Medical Council. *Duties of a doctor: good medical practice*. London: General Medical Council, 1995) stipulates that, as a doctor, you are expected to work constructively within a team, and to respect the skills and contributions of colleagues.

Characteristics of teamwork

- The goals should be discussed and agreed by all members of the team.

- There must be effective communication skills, as these will ensure the free flow of information between team members.

- The relationship between members of the team should be supportive and trusting.

- If disagreement should arise, this should be oriented around the goal, and not directed towards individuals.

- The atmosphere should be non-threatening and non-competitive.

- Team roles should be defined clearly.

As healthcare is increasingly being provided by multidisciplinary teams, working with others is essential for the effective delivery of treatment to patients. Therefore, when applying for a job, team-working skills are a commonly assessed area. The assessment may be through your curriculum vitae, the application form, direct questioning during the interview, or observed group exercises. In order to succeed, you must be able both to show an understanding of the qualities of a good team player and to demonstrate situations where you have shown good team-working skills.

Characteristics of successful team workers

- They treat others with respect.

- They are willing to help.

- They are flexible and open to taking on ideas that differ from their own.

- They demonstrate good communication skills and good listening skills.

- They are reliable.

- They are responsible for their own contributions within the team.

Roles within a team

Different people within a team will contribute in different ways, and to different extents. You must understand your own role within the team, as well as that of others. To do that, you must appreciate all the different roles that people can take in a team.

Having an understanding of the qualities and structures important to the successful working of a team will enable you to identify and portray the qualities that you possess relevant to this section of the application form. You can also then understand how and why your role fits into the overall successful functioning of the team.

Action-oriented roles

- *Shaper*: challenges the team to improve.
- *Implementer*: puts ideas into motion.
- *Completer–finisher*: ensures thorough completion and sticks to deadlines.

People-oriented roles

- *Coordinator*: also known as a chairperson.
- *Team worker*: encourages cooperation.
- *Resource investigator*: explores outside opportunities.

Thought-oriented roles

- *Plant*: presents new ideas and approaches.
- *Evaluator*: analyses the options.
- *Specialist*: provides specialist skills.

 It is easy, but incorrect, to answer a teamwork question by using the words 'team', 'team worker', and 'team working' as many times as possible, but at the same time failing to clearly define your role within that team. If, for example, you were the team leader, ensure that you make this clear.

Leadership skills

Working in the healthcare profession, you will have to adapt to many different situations. Simply being a good team player may not be enough to succeed in the working environment, or during job applications. One day you may take on a passive role within a team, for example writing notes during a ward round, but then you may have to take the lead with junior colleagues, such as during teaching sessions. Leadership skills, therefore, are as important as team-working skills.

Qualities of a successful leader

- Has clear objectives for the task in hand, and is able to communicate and delegate these to the team.

- Sets an example to the rest of the group.

- Is familiar with members of the team, and knows how to motivate each of them.

- Has effective communication skills, including listening skills.

- Has the ability to make decisions.

- Is open to suggestions from other team members, and understands the need for change.

Leadership styles

Within the NHS, as in many organizations, different leadership styles exist and are used in different situations. Which leadership style to adopt at any one time will be suggested by the feedback from members of the team, feedback from people outside the team, and the results produced.

Autocratic

This is the classic approach, whereby the leader retains as much power over decision-making as possible. Other members are expected to obey orders and are not allowed to have much input.

This method can be used successfully in situations where members are new and untrained, and are not aware of how things should be done. This type of leadership can also be useful if there is limited time during which a task needs to be performed. The downside of this, however, may be low team morale, absenteeism, and a fearful and resentful working environment.

Bureaucratic

This form of leadership is where tasks are performed in accordance with policy and protocols. This is useful when routine tasks are performed repeatedly, or in situations where safety is a major concern. However, it can result in the formation of habits that are hard to deviate from. Also, team members may do only what is expected of them, as they are not encouraged to initiate new ideas or approaches.

Democratic

This is where team members are encouraged to be involved in decision-making. This keeps them informed, and shares the responsibilities between individuals. However, if there are many team members, this approach may not be practical. It may be more efficient for the leader to make the decisions, and saves the leader from feeling that his or her role is being threatened.

Laissez-faire or 'hands off'

Here, the leader provides little or no direction, and all members of the team are given as much freedom as possible. The individuals of the team are encouraged to set goals, make decisions, and resolve problems on their own. This is particularly useful if everyone is at a similar level of skill and experience. Therefore, if there are less experienced, more junior members of the team, this will not be successful.

Factors that influence which leadership style to adopt

- The leader's background (personality, experience, ethics, and values).
- Other team members (personalities, background, and experience).
- The organization (values, philosophy, and concerns).

Responses on the application form

The application form questions relating to team working and leadership are considered below and examples are given in the homework section at the end of the chapter. The aim of these questions is to determine whether you are aware of the qualities of a successful teamworker and leader, and can understand the differences between the two. The questions may also ask you to demonstrate, with examples, situations where you have displayed these skills or identified them in others. These questions may relate to your medical training so far, or may be broader and ask for examples from other areas of your life, such as sporting activities.

When answering these questions, the SPAR framework can be used ('Situation, Problem, Action, Result/reflection/relevance' – see Chapter 4). For example, if asked to describe a situation where you worked successfully as part of a team, your question should be structured as follows:

S   What team you were part of? Where was this team based?
P   What were the goals of the team? What was your own role?
A   How did you go about achieving this goal, both personally and as a team?
R   What was the end result, and how did this affect others? What did you learn from this experience, and how is this relevant to Foundation training?

Suitable examples

Application forms for medical school and beyond are obviously based around medical themes. However, they do sometimes ask about your outside interests. Of relevance to teamwork and leadership might be: sporting achievements, interests in the arts (music, painting, etc.), charity work, and business experience. The same principles and structure can be used when answering these questions.

Q: What non-clinical examples can I use when answering a teamwork or leadership question?

A: You can use any experience where you have achieved a quantifiable outcome and where you have learnt skills that are relevant to Foundation training. Here are some examples:
- sporting events and experiences
- public performances (e.g. concerts)
- research projects
- charity fundraising
- events at medical school (e.g. summer ball)
- business ideas
- expeditions
- jobs (outside medicine).

Relevance to the Foundation Programme

The Foundation Programme helps to bridge the gap between medical school and specialist training. The aims are to help you develop skills and interests that will be of benefit to you in deciding and embarking on your career subspecialty. Your medical school should provide you with the knowledge base with which to proceed, but does not always prepare you fully for the duties and responsibilities expected of you as a junior doctor. The application form helps employers differentiate those applicants who will be able to fit into the working environment with the least amount of friction. It is clear why assessing team-working and leadership skills is of importance from the employer's point of view. In order to succeed, you must demonstrate an understanding of these areas, and make yourself appeal to others as somebody with whom they would enjoy working.

Example questions and answers

Q1: Discuss a situation when you successfully worked within a team. (150 words)

Poor answer

During my surgical attachment in my final year of medical school, I sat in during the pre-assessment clinic. A 70-year-old man was to come in for a hernia repair the following week. Of significance, he had a pacemaker.

We weren't sure what to do, and so the F1 doctor I was shadowing asked the registrar. He instructed us to inform the anaesthetist, but as the clinic was extremely busy we didn't have time. I decided to document clearly in the notes that this man was for anaesthetic review, and then left the notes in the consultant anaesthetist's office.

The anaesthetist arranged a review and some other checks and, as far as we know, the operation went ahead without any complications.

Better answer

During my surgical attachment in my final year of medical school, I sat in during the pre-assessment clinic. A 70-year-old man was to come in for a hernia repair the following week. Of significance, he had a pacemaker.

The F1 doctor I was shadowing made an initial assessment, and informed the anaesthetist who would be performing the list. I then took on the task of booking the man for anaesthetic review the following day. I also involved the cardiology registrar, who would need to see the patient to identify the type of pacemaker.

The F1 doctor informed our registrar and consultant about this patient, and the reviews that we were arranging.

While all this was happening, we continued to update the patient, and he left the clinic with a definite follow-up plan to see the relevant specialists. His operation went ahead successfully the following week, and he went on to make a good recovery.

Good answer

I spent 4 years as an active member of my university cricket club, playing and as social secretary and alumni officer. I progressed to a more competitive level of playing at a major county cricket club (Middlesex Under-21s).

As the central part of a squad of 20 cricketers, I was elected captain and led my team to the finals of the University of London cricket championships. I was one of eight in our club to be awarded 'half sporting colours'. I also organized various sports tours and parties, and designed a cricket blazer unique to our club.

The skills I learnt, such as keeping our team together, particularly during losing streaks, ensuring that the strengths of individual members were employed when needed, and boosting team morale with social events, will all be useful when I commence as a Foundation trainee.

Q2: Describe a situation (clinical or non-clinical) where you showed leadership. (150 words)

Model answer

On my medical student elective, I organized a project in Malaysia assessing left ventricular function intraoperatively following cardioplegia. I put the proposal together, secured funding from a national organization, and, with the help of my local supervisor, arranged for a portable ultrasound machine to be available in theatre.

During the project, I taught myself how to operate the machine, and then educated a trainee radiographer in its workings, who became the lead intraoperative ultrasonographer after I left Malaysia. I liaised with the local clinical trial team to collate the necessary data, and, with their help and support, put together a paper that was presented nationally and internationally.

From this experience, I learnt how to coordinate a complex project, mentor a more junior trainee, and take projects to completion with the help and support of an entire team, all skills relevant to Foundation training.

Q1: Discuss a situation in which you successfully worked within a team.

Q2: Describe an example from your own experience (either clinical or non-clinical) that has increased your understanding of the importance of team working. What was your role and contribution to the team?

Q3: Give an example of how you have solved a complex problem through teamwork. What did you learn from this experience?

Q4: Describe a situation (clinical or non-clinical) in which you showed leadership.

Q5: What leadership skills have you acquired during your training?

10 Professional integrity

Philip J Smith

'To thine own self be true' (Polonius, from Shakespeare's *Hamlet*) was often thought to be a suitable definition of the ethos of integrity. A contemporary definition of professional integrity in a clinical setting is 'the ability to do the right thing when faced with a situation that would be easier to ignore'. On application scoring sheets, professional integrity is often summarized as 'the capacity to take responsibility for your own actions and to demonstrate respect for all'.

Professional integrity is arguably one of the most important attributes of any doctor or health professional. The general public want to believe that their doctors are prepared to do the 'right and honest thing' when faced with difficult clinical scenarios. Indeed, demonstrating that you can act with probity is of paramount importance in both medical application forms and interviews, and is one of the major areas in which your character is being tested. Foundation schools can also test your knowledge of clinical governance issues within this sphere, from incident reporting to your understanding of the culture of openness in medical institutions.

Questions on professional integrity

Probity is one of the key features of the GMC's guidance on *Good Medical Practice* (www.gmc-uk.org/guidance/good_medical_practice/index.asp), and is a favourite question on application forms. Such questions can relate to:

119

- a scenario with a difficult or failing colleague
- a deficiency in your own knowledge or training
- patient confidentiality
- communication problems, and acting as a patient's advocate
- mistakes (linked closely to clinical governance issues and the reporting of critical incidents).

To score full marks, you will have to show that you have taken full responsibility for your own actions, demonstrating clear respect for all, and consistently acting within professional boundaries. A deficiency in one of these areas will mean that you will get a lower mark.

Questions that are typically used in application forms do not vary greatly, with most testing your safety, your awareness of ethical principles, and issues surrounding patient confidentiality and consent. Most seek to allow you to demonstrate that you can take responsibility for your actions. Often the questions will have a word limit; therefore, as space is limited, you need to make the best use of it.

Common pitfalls to avoid

- **Defining an action as 'professional integrity' when it isn't.**

- **Making yourself look more professional than another colleague.**

- **Laying blame on an individual.**

- **Dealing with complex situations on your own, that is, without consulting a senior colleague or another member of the multidisciplinary team.**

- **Not considering the feelings of the patient or person concerned.**

- **Dangerous mistakes (e.g. stating that you accidentally injected someone with 10 times the correct dose of morphine will endear you only to the medical defence lawyers!).**

Responses using structured techniques

The questions presented in the online application form are generally best answered using the structured SPAR approach ('Situation, Problem, Action, Result/reflection/relevance' – see Chapter 4). An example is given below.

Q1: Describe one example of a recent clinical situation in which you demonstrated appropriate professional behaviour. What did you do, and what did you learn? How will you apply this to Foundation training? (150 words)

Model answer

[Situation]
During my oncology attachment, I clerked a patient in accident and emergency with metastatic cancer whose family were unaware of her diagnosis. Later, an anxious and hostile relative approached me, demanding to know what her diagnosis was.

[Problem, Action]
Concerned about breaking the patient's confidentiality, I calmly and politely explained I was a medical student, and would not be able to discuss this with them without her consent, but suggested that they speak with the patient together with the consultant in charge of her care if necessary. I remained calm throughout, trying to reassure and empathically listen to their concerns, and later informed a member of the team of this conversation.

[Reflection]
As a Foundation trainee, I will often be the first point of contact with relatives. This experience taught me to act with integrity through recognizing the limits of my knowledge and competence, maintaining confidentiality, and being sensitive to the needs of relatives.

This is a common situation for a medical student to be placed in. Here, a good candidate has demonstrated several qualities.

Q: *How can I score highly on questions relating to professional integrity?*

A: You must show that you:
- have an awareness of confidentiality and patient autonomy issues
- have the ability to remain calm under pressure
- know when to refer cases to senior colleagues for help
- can suggest possible options to resolve problems
- can take responsibility for your actions
- can learn from your experiences to improve your practice.

COCKUPS

Another common situation to be in either as a medical student or as a Foundation trainee is to be involved in or to witness a clinical mistake or incident. Remember, no one is infallible, and all doctors make mistakes from time to time. What is important, though, is how you respond to and deal with the mistakes that you (or others) have made. Remember, the priority is to make sure that the patient is safe, and then to report the incident, even if it is you who has made the mistake. This is the essence of professional integrity.

When structuring the answer you can still use the SPAR technique, but, when approaching the A and R sections, a useful acronym to remember is COCKUPS:

- *Correct* the mistake; make the situation good once again
- *Open* and transparent approach throughout
- *Critical* incident form/report
- *Keep* professional and be non-judgemental at all times
- *Understand* and learn from the mistake
- *Personal* role, responsibility, reflection
- *Senior* involvement (always!).

Q2: Describe a situation where you were aware that a mistake occurred in the workplace. What did you do, and how did this influence the outcome? (150 words)

Good answer 1

[Situation, Problem]
A patient with multiple myeloma presented to the day unit generally unwell and requiring hospital admission. The F1 doctor I was shadowing was asked to check the patient's blood results by the haematology consultant. Later that day, we checked the results, but accidentally overlooked the result showing a corrected calcium of 3.7.

[Action]
The next day I discovered this result, and immediately informed the F1 doctor, who started intravenous fluids and bisphosphonate treatment. We apologized to the patient for the delay and both of us informed the team specialist registrar, who sensitively asked the F1 doctor what had happened, explaining that no one was infallible, and supporting him in a non-accusatory manner. We informed the consultant, completing a clinical incident form together, in an open and honest way, maintaining our integrity.

[Reflection]
We presented this scenario to the trust clinical governance board, suggesting that the on-call team be informed about all significantly abnormal biochemistry results. This was accepted as trust policy.

Good answer 2

[Situation, Problem]
I sat in on the gastroenterology outpatient clinic with the registrar and saw a patient with weight loss and dyspepsia who required an OGD. Assisting the registrar, I completed the endoscopy request form, giving it to the patient to take to the endoscopy suite, while the registrar moved on to see the next patient. Later I realized that I had ticked the box on the form saying that the patient needed bowel preparation as for a colonoscopy.

[Action]
I immediately informed the registrar of my error, who rang the patient to explain and apologize for my mistake, ensuring that she understood not to take the bowel preparation. We reported my mistake to the consultant and completed a critical incident form in an open and transparent manner.

[Reflection]
On reflection, we recommended to the trust that the prescription forms for colonoscopy and OGD be on separate sheets, so similar mistakes could not occur.

Poor answer

A patient with multiple myeloma presented to the day unit generally unwell and requiring hospital admission. The F1 doctor I was shadowing was asked to check the patient's blood results by the haematology consultant. Later that day, we forgot to check the test results as we were busy on the wards, overlooking the result showing a corrected calcium of 3.7.

The next day I discovered this result, and informed the same F1 doctor, who advised that I call the on-call F1 as he was off duty now. I handed over to the nursing staff to ring the team specialist registrar to inform him the F1 had missed the results. He then left his outpatient clinic to see the patient. The angry specialist registrar later asked the F1 what had happened, and asked why it had taken so long for the patient's treatment to be started. He informed the consultant and completed a clinical incident form.

Later that day, the F1 rang the biochemistry laboratory to ask why they had not informed them of the result, explaining that this was unacceptable and that they would be held accountable if anything were to happen to the patient.

The example above is similar to the previous model answer but paints the F1 doctor in a very bad light (even if it is true) and apportions blame. Furthermore, the answer does not demonstrate clearly that the candidate has taken responsibility nor immediately made the patient safe (the first priority). A candidate with this sort of answer would score poorly on the professional integrity part of the application form.

Therefore, as with all the other sections, it is worth sitting down for a considerable amount of time and thinking of good examples from your training that can be used to answer the question. Remember, the answer has to be believable, and must demonstrate your understanding and appreciation of the principles and importance of probity.

- Remember the common pitfalls.
- Use the SPAR technique in your answers.
- Remember COCKUPS for mistakes.
- Fail to prepare and you prepare to fail, so practise, practise, practise!

Q1: Describe one example of a recent clinical situation where you demonstrated appropriate professional behaviour. What did you do, and what have you learned? How will you apply this to Foundation training?

Q2: Describe a situation in which you were aware that a mistake occurred in the workplace. What did you do, and how did this influence the outcome?

Q3: Describe an example of a situation in which you had to demonstrate your professionalism and/or integrity. What did you do, and what was the outcome?

11 The patient as the central focus of care

Mark J Portou, Manoj Ramachandran, and Marc A Gladman

Modern medical graduates must possess, and then demonstrate, a broad range of essential skills and competences in order to be successful in their careers. In addition to the numerous non-clinical skills (e.g. teamwork, leadership, and professionalism) that have already been covered, clinical skills are crucial for Foundation doctors, particularly the ability to place the patient as the central focus of care in all given situations.

All patients have needs. By virtue of being assessed and treated by physicians and surgeons, these individuals have assumed a 'sick role', and thus are in a vulnerable position. When answering any question on patients, it is important to consider their care in the context of their *physical–psychological–social–spiritual* needs. This approach is termed holistic care.

> **Patients' needs can be divided into:**
>
> - physical
> - psychological
> - social
> - spiritual.

Most applicants will choose to detail a patient's physical needs in their response to the question on the application form relating to patient care, although some may choose mental health problems or needs. However, it is crucial not to fail to address the non-physical needs of the patient. These are considered in turn, below.

Physical needs

The physical needs of any patient may include:

- analgesia
- antibiotics
- surgery
- high-dependency/intensive care
- resuscitation.

This is not an exhaustive list, and any medical intervention is likely to be aimed at addressing a physical need and is thus relevant.

Psychological needs

Psychological needs may not be immediately obvious, but will have an enormous impact on the patient's wellbeing if not addressed. Dealing with these issues may simply require reassurance and letting the patient express any fears; in more extreme instances, however, pharmacological agents may be required, such as antidepressants.

The psychological issues that patients have may include:

- depression
- institutionalization
- fear of dying
- loss of function/purpose
- loss of confidence.

Social needs

The patient's social needs include not only home circumstances. The long-term effects of illness and prolonged hospital stays also have to be addressed. Dealing with the social needs of a patient requires a truly multidisciplinary approach, and involves engagement with professionals allied to medicine, such as nursing staff, occupational therapists, physiotherapists, and social workers.

The social issues that patients may have include:

- burden of chronic disease

- effect on family and relationships

- financial

- dependants (e.g. patient as main carer for spouse)

- the need for home assistance.

Spiritual needs

The spiritual issues that a patient may have include:

- effect of religion/beliefs as a comforting influence

- loss of faith.

Learning points and reflection

It may sound clichéd, but every patient encounter is a learning experience. It is, therefore, crucial to explain to the scorer the educational benefit obtained from the individual examples that you have chosen in your answer. It cannot be emphasized often enough that *all* questions on the application form require reflection, and an explanation of both what was learned from the experience and how this will make you a better Foundation Programme doctor.

Learning points from patient encounters with direct relevance to the Foundation Programme include:

- specific knowledge of disease management

- role of multidisciplinary team

- communication skills observed and practised

- breaking bad news

- holistic approach in action.

Example question and answers

Compare and contrast the care pathways that you have observed for two different patients with similar clinical problems. To what extent did each pathway take the individual needs of the patient into account? What have you learnt from these patients that will be relevant to your Foundation training? (250 words)

In contrast to the other responses, a word limit of 250 words was available for the response to this question on the 2008 form.

Q: *What is a 'care pathway'?*

A: In this context, the term 'care pathways' refers to the patient's journey or experience. It encompasses all events from presentation and admission to hospital right through to discharge. It should not be confused with formal 'care pathways', which in many hospitals are in place to standardize the management of common medical conditions, such as asthma or diabetic ketoacidosis.

Q: *How should I break this question down when planning my response?*

A: This is a complex question, with numerous components. You should consider each of the following:
1. Identify two different patients with similar problems but managed in different ways ('care pathways').
2. Identify each patient's needs (physical–psychological–social–spiritual).
3. Compare and contrast each pathway, considering their effects on the patient.
4. Explain what you have learned, having been involved with these different approaches.
5. Explain how this will be relevant to your Foundation training.

For this answer, you must briefly describe from your own experience *two* separate patients with *similar diseases or even the same disease*. You must then briefly describe similarities and/or differences in their 'care pathways'. You must then identify, and comment on, how far these patients had their 'needs' met. Finally, you should state what you learned from these patients, and how this new-found knowledge/experience would benefit your Foundation training.

Poor answer

During a placement on a liver transplant unit, I observed the care of two patients with cirrhosis secondary to alcoholic liver disease. The first patient was a publican in his late forties, who presented acutely with ascites, jaundice, and encephalopathy. He underwent a CT of his abdomen, which showed a scarred liver, consistent with cirrhosis. This man was treated with a paracentesis to drain the ascites, and given terlipressin to reduce portal venous pressures and help reduce the risk of variceal bleeding. His encephalopathy was treated with lactulose, and raised INR with intravenous vitamin K. He survived this episode of decompensation and was eventually discharged home, having also been treated for alcohol withdrawal.

The second patient, a man in his sixties, had been abstinent for around six months, and was on the liver transplant waiting list. He was admitted from clinic with worsening ascites for paracentesis, which he had on a regular basis due to its rapid reaccumulation, despite the use of diuretics. This patient went home the next day after the drain was removed. A donor liver was eventually found, and he underwent a successful liver transplantation. Observing the management of these two patients has made me more confident in managing patients with liver disease.

This answer gives two different examples, but, rather than comparing and contrasting the two care pathways, the candidate merely describes each of the patients and his treatment in turn. The answer offers no reflection and, although the use of medical jargon may sound impressive, there is little evidence of any learning from these patients. No discussion is given of the care pathways, and no relevance to the Foundation Programme is identified. This answer would thus score very poorly.

Better answer

> *During my final-year medicine placement, I encountered two diabetic patients, an elderly woman with long-standing poorly controlled type 2 diabetes, and a young woman presenting with diabetic keto-acidosis. The management of these patients utilized multidisciplinary team input, and required similar investigations and insulin-based treatments to be commenced.*
>
> *For the elderly patient, the diabetic nurse specialist was crucial to her in-patient care and, through regular education, advice, and training sessions, her poor compliance with medication and unsuitable diet were addressed. Conversely, the care of the young woman focused on the acute management of a medical emergency, with early specialist input and utilization of the critical-care outreach services. Once stable, the diabetic multidisciplinary team, including the specialist diabetologist, dietician, and pharmacists, were able to educate and reassure this patient, answer her questions, provide support following her initial diagnosis, and institute a tailored insulin regimen.*
>
> *From these contrasting examples, I learnt that common chronic conditions such as diabetes may have similar medical treatments, but the delivery of care differs greatly, and must be tailored to the individual patient, utilizing an effective multidisciplinary team.*

This answer is much better than the previous example. Although it can be argued that type 1 and type 2 diabetes are not the same disease, they are probably similar enough for the purposes of this example. The patients are described well, and a clear contrast is provided. However, it remains uncertain whether the needs of the individual patients were met. Some evidence of reflection in the last paragraph is apparent, but no clear evidence of learning or relevance to the Foundation Programme is provided. This answer started well and promised much, but unfortunately finished weakly.

Good answer

While a student in a regional cardiothoracic centre, I observed the care of two men admitted electively for pulmonary lobectomy, as definitive management for lung carcinoma. These patients both had extensive smoking histories. The first patient presented with shortness of breath and weight loss, and had multiple co-morbidities. In contrast, the second patient was fit and well, and was diagnosed incidentally on a routine chest X-ray. This man had difficulty accepting his diagnosis, and worried about losing employment and the subsequent financial burden on his family. He benefited from early input from Macmillan nurse specialists, who helped to address his social and psychological concerns.

The postoperative recovery of both was complicated by pain, requiring anaesthetic input, and for the first patient intercostal nerve blocks. The second patient, through early mobilization with physiotherapists, quickly regained his confidence, and was discharged on the sixth postoperative day. The first patient unfortunately developed pneumonia, requiring intravenous antibiotics, and was later intubated and managed on ITU. He was eventually discharged home following rehabilitation with the occupational therapists and physiotherapists.

From these patients, I learnt the importance of a holistic and multidisciplinary approach to the care of surgical patients. This experience reiterated the roles of the healthcare professionals whom I will be working alongside and learning from as a Foundation trainee. I also learnt the importance of effective pain control and fluid balance when managing patients postoperatively, and observed the escalation of treatment required in acutely sick patients. I will consolidate and expand on this knowledge and experience during my Foundation training.

This worked example is structured using the SPAR technique (see Chapter 4), and concisely and clearly describes two different patients with the same disease. It addresses the different needs of each patient, and explains how they were resolved using contrasting methods. The example also shows evidence of reflection and learning from these experiences, and importantly demonstrates the relevance to Foundation training.

Q1: Compare and contrast the care pathways you have observed for two different patients with similar clinical problems. To what extent did each pathway take the individual needs of the patient into account? What have you learnt from these patients that will be relevant to your Foundation training?

Q2: Describe an example from your clinical experience where your behaviour enhanced the experience of the patient as the central focus of care. What did you do, and what was the outcome.

12 Teaching, learning, audit, and research

Jasdeep Gill

The Department of Health has introduced a 'lifelong learning' framework, which primarily aims to support staff in the acquisition of new skills, and to ensure that patients benefit from a better-qualified and more motivated workforce. Commitment to lifelong learning is an acknowledgement that becoming professionally qualified is merely the beginning of a career. Regularly updating skills and knowledge as part of your continuing professional development is essential to career progression, particularly given the passing of the concept of a 'job for life', and redefined career pathways.

Lifelong learning can take place any time and anywhere, as long as your mind is open to the experience. It is broadly divided into formal and informal learning. Informal learning describes learning that is unplanned. Formal learning refers to the scheduled teaching that you attend. As part of your Foundation training, you will be required to keep a log in your learning portfolio of both formal and informal learning. For example, as reflective summaries in your portfolio, you should keep a log of interesting cases you see, and identify the key learning points as evidence of informal learning. It is worth getting into good habits early: start doing this now for interesting patients you see on the wards.

The introduction of learning portfolios and competency-based training further emphasizes the drive towards lifelong learning.

However, it also demonstrates the shift from the 'teacher as expert', which involved a didactic teaching approach, to the 'teacher as facilitator', which involves a teacher guiding the learner towards sources of knowledge so that the learner discovers the answer. Teaching styles that support this approach include problem-based learning (PBL), self-directed learning (SDL), and discussion. Many medical schools have a mixture of teaching styles within their courses. From the descriptions below, try to identify which is the predominant teaching style for you.

Teaching and learning styles

Didactic/direct instruction

This is the traditional, teacher-centred approach. The teacher provides the learner with the majority of the information required, often via lectures. This style allows minimal teacher–learner interaction and requires supplementation by examples, practice, and discussion to check understanding.

Discussion

This involves interactive and free dialogue between the teacher and learner. It involves more than simply a question–answer period, because it requires the teacher to give control to the learners to express their thoughts. It requires open-mindedness and mutual respect between the teacher and learner.

Problem-based learning

This involves learning through structured exploration of a research problem. Learners work in small groups to define, carry out, and reflect upon a research task, which can often be a 'real-life' scenario, using a systematic approach. The teacher acts as a facilitator to whom the learner can turn for guidance.

Self-directed learning/instruction

This is a learner-centred approach. It allows learners to take responsibility for their own learning by applying their knowledge to real-life scenarios, monitoring their own achievement, and exploring sources for further information. It encourages the learner to apply independent thinking, and enhances the development of reasoning, judgement, and critical thinking.

Competence-based questions

Maintaining good learning and teaching practices not only helps you in your day-to-day role as a doctor, but is also excellent for building up your curriculum vitae (on which, see Chapter 13). Employers are keen to see your skills in teaching, appraisal, and mentorship, and so the Foundation Programme application questions will ask for specific examples of your ability or experience in a particular area. This style of questioning is termed 'competence based'. Competence-based questions allow candidates to demonstrate that they possess the skills that are necessary for the job.

 When answering competence-based questions, it is better to use specific examples rather than to write broadly about your general experiences.

With lifelong learning and continuing professional development being so high on the healthcare agenda, there is no doubt that there will be questions relating to your academic achievements and teaching experience on the Foundation application form. Below are some worked examples of Foundation application questions. Each question has been broken down and answered twice, first with an example of a poor answer and then with an example of a better answer, using the SPAR technique (see Chapter 4) where applicable.

You must remember that the advice given is only an example to get you thinking. and to offer you some guidance. Also remember *never to lie, fabricate, or plagiarize*, regardless of how tempting it may seem. Even aligning your answers to the examples in this book is asking for trouble. Your Foundation school could ask for verification of your answers, so ensure that your paperwork and certificates are in order.

Example questions and answers

Q1: Describe one example of a teaching session you conducted and the teaching style you used. What did you learn, and how will you apply this to your Foundation training? (150 words)

This question has many parts, so start off by breaking it down and highlighting the key words. Notably this question is about teaching, teaching styles, and your experience of teaching. It goes on to ask for reflection on what you learnt, and its application to your subsequent training. Even if the question did not directly ask for this, you should aim to complete your answer with a sentence or two of reflection. Always keep referring back to the question as you write your answer, to ensure that you respond to each component of the question.

Move on next to think about potential examples of teaching that you could use. This could be in relation to your medical training or any other experience, such as teaching medical students in lower years (e.g. examination skills, clinical skills, basic life support classes), teaching schoolchildren (e.g. health education), or teaching in any extracurricular area in which you are skilled (e.g. sports, cookery, dance). Whichever example you use, be clear and concise in your description. Remember, you will be marked on how you taught and your experience, rather than exactly whom and what you taught. Aim to show some insight into why you chose the teaching methods that you used. When teaching any audience or group, feedback is always a useful component to help your future performance, so you should aim to mention this in your answer.

Poor answer

During summer this year I taught a group of third-year medical students suturing skills. They had identified that this was a topic they wished to learn about. As a member of the university Surgical Society, I had attended suturing sessions, which I found to be useful and wanted to pass on the skills I had learnt.

I booked a clinical skills room and organized the equipment required for the practical part of the teaching session. I talked the students through the principles of suturing using a PowerPoint presentation and then supervised them while they practised.

The students provided positive feedback and approved of my teaching technique. I refreshed and enhanced my suturing skills, which will be useful during the surgery part of Foundation training.

This answer is superficial and waffles at the start. It describes how the teaching was done but demonstrates that the candidate does not have insight into teaching styles. The final sentence correctly reflects on what the candidate learnt; however, it demonstrates that the candidate has misidentified the point of this question.

Better answer

I taught health education to classes of 12–14 year olds with a colleague. The school identified the curriculum, which included physical, mental, and sexual health topics.

I attended an intensive 4-week training and teaching skills programme. I devised a timetable for the sessions, and incorporated a mixture of didactic teaching alongside discussion and self-directed learning, which created a balance and maintained the students' interest. I encouraged student participation, summarized salient points, and used a quiz to check their understanding.

This experience significantly increased my confidence in public speaking. I learnt to absorb technical information and convey it simply with a logical flow. I will demonstrate these skills during Foundation training when educating patients to maximize their understanding and satisfaction.

This experience improved my ability to work alongside a colleague and accept constructive criticism. This will enable me to reflect on feedback positively to improve my performance during Foundation training.

This answer covers each component of the question and works through the SPAR approach. The use of buzzwords such as 'didactic' and 'self-directed learning' illustrates that the candidate has knowledge of teaching styles. The answer demonstrates that the candidate recognizes teaching as a fundamental component of patient care and has identified that patient education, understanding, and satisfaction are essential. The final paragraph adds further depth to the answer, with more reflection on the skills learnt and their relevance to Foundation training.

Q2: Describe one example of research or audit from your undergraduate medical training. What was your role, and what contribution did you make? What did you learn, and how will you apply this to your Foundation training? (150 words)

It is important to understand the difference between research and audit. Research is an attempt to determine generalizable new knowledge by addressing clearly definable questions with systematic and rigorous methods. Audit, on the other hand, is a quality process that seeks to improve patient care and outcomes through systematic review of care against explicit criteria and the implementation of change. To put it simply, research tells us what we should be doing, while audit tells us how well we are doing it.

To start off, break down the question and identify the key words within it. This question focuses on your experience of research or audit. It specifically asks for your role and contribution, and so you must answer this directly. Wrap up your answer by identifying what you learnt, and its application to your Foundation training.

Carefully consider which research or audit project to use as an example. If you have conducted only one piece during your undergraduate medical training, then you can use only that example. However, if you have several under your belt, you should aim to use the one in which you had greatest involvement, even if its outcome was less significant.

Most pieces of research or audit are conducted as part of a team, and so it is important that you clearly identify the extent of your involvement. If, on the other hand, you conducted it single-handedly, then you must say so – this is not a time for modesty. Identify your role clearly and concisely. When describing your role, be careful not to display other colleagues in a poor light to make yourself look better. Use power verbs to portray your contribution.

Q: *What are good examples of power verbs to use in the application?*

A: A selection of useful power verbs is given below:
- accomplished
- coordinated
- designed
- directed
- established
- evaluated
- facilitated
- formulated
- negotiated
- organized
- prioritized
- scheduled
- supervised
- validated.

Poor answer

I studied diabetes self-management on a group of 200 patients using an anonymized questionnaire. This large-scale study was conducted by myself and a colleague.

I took initiative to set up the research, and applied for and secured ethical approval. My colleague designed the questionnaire, which I printed and piloted on 20 patients. We achieved approval from the diabetes consultant. As primary researchers, my colleague and I undertook the data collection and we liaised with the reception staff and diabetes nurses to aid in the distribution and collection of the questionnaires. Their assistance was forthcoming, and between us we achieved 100% uptake of the questionnaires. We analysed the data together and performed statistical analysis.

Our findings were significant and we successfully published the research in the Journal of Diabetes.

This answer is too narrative. Although the question asks for your role and contribution, it does not ask for a running commentary. There is excessive use of 'we' and 'our', which makes the reader question how much the candidate really contributed. Avoid lying or fabricating at all costs, but if you did something, then say so clearly. Furthermore, in this answer there is no reflection on what the candidate learnt or its application to Foundation training. This means that one-third of the question has not been answered, and so a third of the marks available have been lost. Make sure that you always keep referring to the question as you write your answer, to ensure that you address each of its components.

Better answer

I noted an inappropriately high use of clopidogrel during my general practice attachment, contrary to the guidelines. Following discussion with my GP supervisor, I initiated and managed an audit of the use of clopidogrel.

I defined the standards following a literature search, and designed a pro forma for data collection, which I performed myself using the computerized patient records. I conducted the data analysis, which demonstrated that almost half of clopidogrel prescriptions were inappropriate. This audit led to multidisciplinary teaching and greater awareness of the guidelines. I completed the audit loop after 6 months, and found greater adherence to the guidelines.

I enhanced my project management skills and discovered the importance of audit in improving clinical practice and patient safety. During my Foundation training, I will ensure that guidelines are followed when prescribing any medication and that evidence-based medicine is practised.

This answer concisely addresses every part of the question. The example selected is very well thought out, and clearly demonstrates that the candidate has sound knowledge of the audit cycle. Using an example of audit lends itself well to this question, as candidates can work through the cycle as part of the description of their role and contribution.

The worked examples above should now have you thinking about ways to approach and structure your answers for your Foundation application questions on teaching, learning, research, and audit.

You will be required to contribute to the education of students and colleagues, and to keep your skills and knowledge up to date throughout your career by regularly taking part in educational activities, research, and audit, to improve your practice. Maintaining good medical practice consists of teaching and training alongside your own lifelong learning. As you can see, teaching and learning will be an important part of your career and do not stop at medical school.

Q1: Describe one example of a teaching session you conducted and the teaching style you used. What did you learn, and how will you apply this to your Foundation training?

Q2: Describe one example of research or audit from your undergraduate medical training. What was your role, and what contribution did you make? What have you learned, and how will you apply this to your Foundation training?

13 The curriculum vitae

Philip J Smith and
Manoj Ramachandran

The Latin meaning of curriculum vitae (CV) is *'the course of one's life'*. Despite application forms now dominating the recruitment process for junior doctors, building and maintaining an up-to-date medical curriculum vitae are still crucial. A CV forms the solid basis from which an application form can be tackled. By developing a CV from an early point in your career, you can ensure that you are strong in the various areas of any application form.

Reasons for keeping an up-to-date CV

- Your CV provides the perfect overview of your medical career.

- It helps you to remember the things that you have done, and the order that you have done them in.

- It helps you to identify weaknesses in your career to date, which in turn will allow you to strengthen them.

- You can develop your portfolio of achievements from your CV.

- It can even help you decide which area of medicine is meant for you. For example, if your CV is clearly full of surgically related achievements, then perhaps surgery is for you.

- You can use your CV to impress potential future employers.

In a nutshell, start keeping your CV up to date as soon as possible. If you are reading this and you are in the final year of medical school or in the Foundation years, then start immediately.

General CV tips

- Be consistent – keep everything in reverse chronological or chronological order throughout the CV (i.e. either from past to present or vice versa – but be consistent).

- Do not be afraid to sell yourself – nobody else will.

- Always be truthful.

- Update it constantly.

- Get people to read it, such as your senior colleagues and friends. A good critic can point out important key points that you may have missed.

- In addition, get people outside of medicine to read your CV, to get as many opinions as possible.

Starting out

It is often difficult to know where to start when writing a CV, but a good way is to take some time and write down all the things that you are proud of, and then try to order them under the following headings:

- degrees
- prizes, awards, grants, honours, distinctions
- postgraduate, undergraduate qualifications (e.g. BSc)
- publications
- presentations – local, national, and international
- audits

- teaching – medical students, laypeople, nurses, other health professionals
- courses and conferences attended
- elective details
- extracurricular activities and responsibilities.

You may or may not have something to put under each of these headings. However, by going through this simple process, you will identify the areas that need extra work.

Around these achievements, a CV is also a useful place to document your employment history, clinical skills (and those you aim to learn), and career aspirations.

There is no defined right or wrong way to write a CV, so this chapter merely offers a structure based around various key headings.

Personal details

You should start with a section that sets out your personal details, for example:

Name: Dr Joseph Bloggs
Date of Birth: 22 May 1981
Address: 6 Saxon Green, London E6 4AR
Tel: 0777 889911
Email: bloggs@doctors.org.uk
Nationality: British
GMC number: 1234567
Driving licence: Full

Some people also include a passport photo adjacent to the personal details.

Photos on a CV
As a general rule, it is best *not* to include a photo of yourself on your CV. It can be interpreted in many ways, most of them negative. Ask yourself this simple question: does your photo sell anything about you, your abilities, or your achievements that are relevant to the job for which you are applying? Unless you are applying to a modelling agency, the answer here really should be no!

School education

This can be kept brief, especially if you are several years post-qualification. Most people will not be interested in GCSE and A-level results (or equivalents) after you have been at medical school for 5 or 6 years, which is why you should really consider writing your CV in reverse chronological order. A summary of recent educational history such as secondary school and sixth form is probably enough:

St Paul's Cathedral School, London	1992–1997
10 GCSEs: 7A*s, 1A, 1B	
St Paul's Cathedral College, London	1997–1999
4 A-levels: 4 A grades	
St Bartholomew's Medical School	1999–2006

Degrees

If still at medical school, then any degree classification may be pending, but should be included, in addition to any intercalated degree results:

MBBS (Honours)   July 2006
St Bartholomew's Medical School

BSc in Immunology (first class)   July 2005
University of London

Postgraduate and undergraduate qualifications

This may not be applicable to medical students and F1 doctors, but will become increasingly important throughout your career. Remember, a CV is a dynamic document that will need regular updating and adjustment.

The types of qualifications that you may want to include are undergraduate qualifications such as BSc or BMedSci, and collegiate examinations such as MRCP or MRCS. With the latter, it is important to state the stage of examination that you are in, such as Part 1 or Part 2.

Remember, keep this all in time order (preferably reverse chronological), stating the date of passing the examination.

MRCP Part 1 examination   July 2008
Royal College of Physicians of England

Dates on a CV

Q: *Does it matter when I passed my exams?*

A: It is far more important *that* you passed the exam rather than *when* you took it. As a general rule, *what* you did is more important than *with whom* or *where* you did it, which in turn are more important than *when* you did it.

Prizes and awards

These can be university awards, national or local awards, elective awards, medical school distinctions, study travel awards, competitive essay awards, or even the Duke of Edinburgh awards.

Don't be shy in putting these into your CV – they have been crucial points on recent applications for jobs. Again, keep them in time order, stating the awarding body and the date of the award.

Don't panic if you do not have any of these: the fact that you are even thinking about these now means that you can do something about this.

Boosting the prizes and awards section

- If you are at medical school, ask about essay competitions, and university and travel awards for electives, in your faculty offices, and look on university websites. Awards such as the British Medical and Dental Student Travel (BMDST) Award are popular.

- Visit Royal College websites to see if there are any sections that offer awards or prizes to junior doctors or medical students.

- Search the internet for opportunities available (the website of the British Medical Association, for example, has links for prizes and grants).

Medical school distinctions vary between institutions. Some do not award any, while at others they are commonplace. Do not be despondent if your university does not readily give out awards, but do look for alternatives.

Publications

This is the most stressful section for *everyone*, not just you! This is why thinking about your CV early in your career is a good idea, as having a publication will make you stand out in an application. It is very hard to get even good quality work published, but definitely worth it.

Publication can take many different forms – from whole books or book chapters to case reports, research, audit, or even letters in journals. All of these can be presented under different subheadings.

If you have got them, great! If not, *don't panic*!

Boosting the publication section of your CV

- Think of research projects completed at university, perhaps as part of an intercalated degree, which could lead to a publication.

- Think of an interesting patient on whom you could prepare a case presentation for submission to a journal (perhaps a medical school journal such as the *Student BMJ*).

- Visit the library and look through journals in an area that you are interested in, and see whether they have a section for case reports, or audits. The key is to find an area of interest and then work towards completing something in that area.

- Speak to your more senior colleagues – ask their advice on any projects that you could get involved in, with the aim of getting some of your work published. If they are clinicians, they could even help you set up audit projects and complete them.

- Visit journal websites, look at the guidelines and directions for potential authors, and follow them very closely to avoid unnecessary rejection.

- If you do have work rejected by journals, do not take it personally, and do not let it put you off trying again.

Sometimes you will have started working on a project and submitted it to a journal, but not heard back. In this situation, you can state on a CV that something is currently under submission, referencing it in the standard way (see below, and see also Chapter 5 on referencing).

Referencing

Referencing your work correctly is very important. One standard format for papers in journals is as follows:

Rasher, A. (2007) How much and how often should we eat bacon? *Danish Bacon Journal* **332**: 1224–1225.

For a book the format would be (where Manchester is the place of publication):

Egg, A. and Sausage, A. (2007) *Fried Food: Eat today, die tomorrow,* 3rd edn. Manchester: Lardy Publishing.

If you have published a part of a BSc degree, or a particularly complex research project, it might be useful to put a brief explanation of that research underneath the reference. This is useful if preparing for an interview and you need to provide a concise explanation of the publication.

Remember, always place your publications in time order, and be consistent in their presentation!

Presentations and audits

The majority of people will have done a presentation at some point, on topics such as research, clinical cases, or audit. You can make yours stand out using the following simple structure and subheadings:

- *Local* – under this heading, list presentations that you have made to your firm, or at weekly teaching sessions
- *Regional* – presentations to your local trust, or at regional meetings

- *National* – presentations to a conference or meeting
- *International* – as above, but not in the country where you live!

How to cite a presentation

'Are eggs, bacon, sausages, and mushrooms essential for traditional fried breakfast?', 9th Congress of European Federation of Deep Fat Fryers, Grimsby, England, 23–26 May 2007.

Teaching

It is essential that you include a section in your CV on this, as Modernizing Medical Careers (see Chapter 1) now demands that every doctor shows competence and ability in this arena.

Whether your experience is in teaching medical students, professionals allied to medicine (e.g. nurses), or teaching schoolchildren basic life support, it is important to clearly document it in as many different areas as possible. Alongside this, you can get your students to fill out feedback forms, so that you have *evidence* of your teaching abilities.

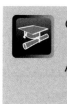

Q: *What is the best type of feedback to demonstrate on my CV or in my portfolio?*

A: You should aim to have evidence of anonymized written feedback from a variety of sources.

Always document whether teaching is done formally or informally, in small or large groups, by problem-based learning (PBL) or topic-based learning, interactively or didactically, or bedside or classroom (and note that these are all key words to use in your CV!). (On teaching and learning styles, see Chapter 12.)

This section is also an opportunity to mention any courses (such as the Teaching TIPS for Teachers Course) that you have done to improve your teaching.

Teaching is a crucial part of medical application forms and interviews, and so it is worth dedicating time to this part of your CV.

Courses

This section is often presented as a list in reverse chronological order. Remember to include here vital courses, such as one on advance life support (ALS). An example listing might be:

Teaching TIPS for Clinical Teachers Course, Royal Free Hospital, London, October 2007

Radiology: Chest and Abdominal Film Interpretation Course, Northwick Park Hospital, London, February 2007

Employment history

This section can be presented in many different ways. However, the most straighforward is to state the specialty, the consultants you worked for, the hospital you worked in, and the dates of your employment there. An example would be:

Endocrinology/General Medicine
Dr G Toms, Newham Hospital, London
August–November 2006

Respiratory Medicine
Dr G Packe, Newham Hospital, London
May–August 2006

Haematology
Dr W Mills/Dr K Zegocki, Newham Hospital, London
February–May 2006

Geriatric/General Medicine
Dr M Britton/Dr B Dasgupta, Homerton Hospital, London
August 2005–February 2006

Clinical skills

This section is often documented in list format, under headings indicating procedures that can be done *independently* (e.g. venepuncture, cannulation) and those that you can undertake *under supervision* (e.g. central line insertion). Skills need to be tailored to expectations for your level of experience (e.g. you probably wouldn't expect an F1 doctor to be able to insert central lines without supervision).

Be as brief as you can with this section, as most trainees at your level will have similar numbers of procedures under their belt. On the other hand, you may appear untrainable if you have performed more procedures than the senior person reading your CV!

Personal responsibilities

This section can be written as prose or presented as bullet points. It demonstrates that you are not frightened of taking on responsibility. Examples such as being the Doctors' Mess President or the MMC/BMA representative may in addition show organizational skills. Remember to state the role that you played when working as a member of a team. This may be very useful when answering application form questions about your ability to handle responsibility.

Extracurricular activities

This is the section in which you can show that you are a well-rounded individual. If these activities also show off your individual attributes, such as leadership, team-working abilities, and organizational skills, so much the better. This is also a good section in which to state exceptional abilities in particular areas, such as in sports or music.

> **Choose very carefully what you put down under extracurricular activities, as it may be misinterpreted. For example, writing 'I have a passion for travelling to exotic places around the world, travelling as much and as often as possible' may be interpreted by some as 'My daddy is extremely wealthy, so I can afford to jet around the world while at medical school', or 'If you want to find me, don't look for me in a lecture theatre – I'm more likely to be found propping up a bar on a beach in Jamaica'. Such a statement may need to be qualified by something to suggest otherwise.**

Elective

If you did something involving a project or won a prize for work achieved on elective, then you could mention it briefly by including this section.

Career aims

The best-written entries here to this will include:

- a plan for the immediate future (gaining competences for the Foundation years, completing a defined research project, performing a specific audit, named courses, etc.)
- a proposed plan for the future (e.g. to take over the world of medicine!).

References

It is important to choose at least two referees, usually your current consultant or educational supervisor, with another consultant of your choice. On your CV, you should state their position, work address, and contact details, once you have ensured that the referee is happy to be just that!

Don't forget ...

You may have the best CV in the world, but, if it looks a mess, it will be binned almost immediately by any prospective employer. You therefore need to consider the following:

- *Font*. Don't use too crazy or eccentric a font. Arial and Times New Roman are most commonly used, with the font size between 10 and 12 points.
- *Length*. At F1/F2 level, aim to get your CV on to three or four pages maximum.
- *Spelling*. You could have the best CV in the world and let youself down by making sily speling and errors grammatical syntax and!

Summary

This chapter has shown you one way of writing a medical CV. Experiment with your CV, and keep writing and rewriting it until you are as happy as you can be with it. It is important to remember the following points:

- Start writing a CV early in your career, and work on the elements that need strengthening.
- Update your CV regularly, as it will be useful for job applications, portfolios, and interviews.
- Always be truthful, but don't be shy about noting your achievements.
- Let people read your CV, as this is the only way you will know how to improve it.

Q1: Write down the top three achievements of your career to date, and define what exactly you achieved in each case (e.g. if you organized an event for charity, how did you do it, and what was the outcome?).

1.

2.

3.

Q2: Write down your short-term and long-term career aims. (You might find it interesting to refer back to this when you update your CV.)

Short-term:

Long-term:

Q3: Write down your extracurricular activities. Try to emphasize the qualities and attributes that sell you as an individual for the job for which you are applying. For example, captaining a volleyball team at university is a good achievement, but leading the team to a great win or keeping the morale of the team going during a losing patch says a lot more about you.

Appendix
Person specification for entry to the Foundation Programme

Adapted from www.foundationprogramme.nhs.uk

	Essential	When it could be evaluated
Eligibility	• Has written approval for this application from the dean (or equivalent) of graduating medical school	Eligibility process/ application
	• Has graduated, or will graduate, from a medical school that is able to provide and validate an academic score	Eligibility process/ application
	• Is fit to practise medicine safely	Eligibility process/ application
	• Has not yet reached the level required for GMC full registration	Eligibility process/ application
	• Has the right to work in the UK which remains valid until 31 July *Or*	Eligibility process/ application
	• Be a student of a UK medical school in the final year of study with existing leave as a student who is available to work in the UK as a doctor from 31 July	Eligibility process/ application
	• Be available to take up the Foundation Programme from 31 July	Eligibility process/ application

	Essential	**When it could be evaluated**
Qualifications	• Has achieved, or is expected to achieve, MBBS or equivalent medical qualification as recognized by the GMC	Eligibility process/ application
	• If previously graduated, will commence programme within 2 years of graduation	Eligibility process/ application
	Or	
	• If graduation will be more than 2 years from commencement of programme, can undergo an assessment to ensure that clinical knowledge and skills have been maintained to the extent that they are appropriate for entry to the Foundation Programme	
Clinical knowledge and skills	• Can demonstrate an understanding and application of good clinical care	Eligibility process/ application Telephone assessment/ pre-employment screening
	• Can demonstrate an understanding and application of maintaining good medical practice	Eligibility process/ application Telephone assessment/ pre-employment screening
	• Can demonstrate an understanding and application of teaching and training, appraising and assessing	Eligibility process/ application Telephone assessment/ pre-employment screening
	• Can demonstrate an understanding and application of relationships with patients	Eligibility process/ application Telephone assessment/ pre-employment screening

	Essential	When it could be evaluated
	• Can demonstrate an understanding and application of working with colleagues	Eligibility process/ application Telephone assessment/ pre-employment screening
	• Can demonstrate an understanding of the outcomes to be achieved and how these are applied in the Foundation Programme as set out in *Tomorrow's Doctors* (2003) (www.gmc-uk.org)	Eligibility process/ application Telephone assessment/ pre-employment screening
Language skills	• Have demonstrable skills in written and spoken English that are adequate to enable effective communication about medical topics with patients and colleagues, which could be demonstrated by either of the following criteria: (a) applicants have undertaken their entire undergraduate medical training in English; *Or* (b) have attained the minimum International English Language Testing System (IELTS) score Minimum scores: Overall 7.5, speaking 7.5, listening 7.5, reading 7.5, writing 7.5.	Eligibility process/ application Pre-employment screening
Personal skills	• Demonstrates an understanding of the importance of the patient as the central focus of care	Application/ pre-employment screening Telephone assessment
	• Demonstrates ability to prioritize tasks and information appropriately	Application/pre-employment screening Telephone assessment

	Essential	When it could be evaluated
	• Demonstrates an understanding of the importance of working effectively with others	Application/ pre-employment screening Telephone assessment
	• Demonstrates the ability to communicate effectively with both colleagues and patients	Application/ pre-employment screening Telephone assessment
	• Demonstrates initiative and the ability to deal effectively with pressure and/or challenge	Application/ pre-employment screening Telephone assessment
Probity	• Demonstrates appropriate professional behaviour, i.e. integrity, honesty, confidentiality, as set out in *Good Medical Practice* (2006) (www.gmc-uk.org/guidance/good_ medical_practice/index.asp)	Application/ pre-employment screening
	• Criminal records clearance at appropriate level subject to prevailing UK legislation	Application/ pre-employment screening

Index